STO

G.

ALLEN COUNTY PUBLIC LIBRARY

ACPL ITEM
DISCARDED

3 1833 00400

S0-BXD-211

61
Lasser, Terese
Reach to recovery

APR 25 '72

Reach to Recovery

by

TERESE LASSER

and

WILLIAM KENDALL CLARKE

Foreword by ARTHUR I. HOLLEB, M.D.
Senior Vice President for Medical Affairs
and Research, American Cancer Society

Epilogue by WILLIAM M. MARKEL, M.D.
Vice President for Service and Rehabilitation,
American Cancer Society

SIMON AND SCHUSTER · NEW YORK

COPYRIGHT © 1972 BY TERESE LASSER & WILLIAM KENDALL CLARKE
ALL RIGHTS RESERVED
INCLUDING THE RIGHT OF REPRODUCTION
IN WHOLE OR IN PART IN ANY FORM
PUBLISHED BY SIMON AND SCHUSTER
ROCKEFELLER CENTER, 630 FIFTH AVENUE
NEW YORK, NEW YORK 10020

FIRST PRINTING

SBN 671-21181-1
LIBRARY OF CONGRESS CATALOG CARD NUMBER: 70-188501
DESIGNED BY EVE METZ
MANUFACTURED IN THE UNITED STATES OF AMERICA
BY AMERICAN BOOK-STRATFORD PRESS, INC., NEW YORK, N.Y.

The lines on page 108 are reprinted from The Prophet, *by Kahlil Gibran, with permission of the publisher, Alfred A. Knopf, Inc. Copyright 1923 by Kahlil Gibran; renewal coypright 1951 by Administrators C.T.A. of Kahlil Gibran Estate and Mary G. Gibran.*

1647040

To all the Reach to Recovery Volunteers all over the world who have lightened the burden of many, because they cared.

CONTENTS

FOREWORD

Terese Lasser is a truly remarkable lady. For many long years, she fought an uphill battle to bring reassurance to women who have had a breast removed. She knew that in our bosom-oriented culture, the psychological impact of a mastectomy was unparalleled by almost any other kind of surgery. Restoration of appearance and arm function, and adjustment to family, marriage and the community, were not easy without help.

As a breast cancer surgeon, I thought I was doing a pretty good job in providing the "pat on the back," the reassuring "Don't worry, my dear, everything will be like it was before," and providing the name of a local corsetiere who was recommended by a trustworthy patient and seemed to satisfy most patients who reported back. Little did I know!

We physicians tend to guard our patients and protect them from the nonprofessionals. We assign responsibility to physicians, nurses and members of the allied health professions. It has also been our custom to discourage patients from discussing their operations with other patients. Our motivation was good. We believed we were acting in the best interests of the woman who had expressed her confidence in our surgical skills by giving free rein to our judgment while she was under anesthesia.

Back in 1952, Terese Lasser had a mastectomy. During her

recuperation, it became clear to her that not enough was being done for the woman whose life had changed so drastically within the space of a few hours. Through trial and error, she gradually learned how to adapt to her new life style. It was not easy by any means. She learned a basic philosophy, which turned out to be a useful approach to the problems of the mastectomy patient.

For she discovered through personal experience that as a mastectomy patient who had adjusted well to her own operation she could provide psychological assistance to other women on a female-to-female basis. How right she was! All one need do is see the look in the eyes of a recently operated mastectomy patient when she first meets a nicely dressed, active and personable woman who says, "I have had the same operation, you are not alone. Can I help you?"

That was the beginning of Reach to Recovery. Terese Lasser (with collaborator William Kendall Clarke) tells the story fully and movingly in this book. As she propagated the idea during her travels and lectures and from a very small office in Manhattan, the medical world gradually became aware of a new activity on the surgical scene.

I must admit that we physicians do not change our ways easily. This is understandable. We are charged with the enormous responsibility of caring for life and death situations. We become protective because some good samaritans who wish to "help" our patients suffer from psychoneuroses or have a morbid interest in disease or wish to dominate the sick patient by demonstrating their own good health. Over the years, we have raised the caution flag and built a high wall between the patient and the nonprofessional.

Physicians and the American Cancer Society knew that

help was being given to the laryngectomy patient who had lost his voice and wanted to learn to speak again; help was being given to the colostomy patient who had an artificial opening on the abdomen; yet most of us who specialized in breast surgery apparently did not recognize that so much more assistance could be given to the woman who had lost a breast.

If the reader thinks for one moment that our society, for centuries, has *not* been breast conscious, all he need do is refer to the Renaissance poets who characteristically described the "heaving lily-white bosom filled with passion"; or, for a more modern approach, check the centerfold of men's magazines and the newspaper advertisements for avant-garde movies. Even the word "mama" is derived from the breast, which is known scientifically as the mammary gland.

Terese Lasser was aware of these facts of life and extended her initial psychological boost to include special exercises for good arm function, information on proper fit of breast forms and clothing for a normal appearance, shopping services, a letter to husbands, advice for teen-age children and innumerable other support mechanisms for total rehabilitation—and all of this at no cost to the patient. The only expenditure was the time, effort and boundless energy of the author, who pursued her vision as she traveled throughout the United States and the world talking to individual patients and to small and large groups of women who were crying for a special kind of help.

Terese Lasser overcame the obstacles of reluctant acceptance at hospitals, the naysayers who gave nothing but discouragement, impossible travel schedules and the limits of physical tolerance in her one-woman campaign.

Through her determination, the Reach to Recovery Program began to catch on. The more Terese Lasser extended herself, the more one saw the women she had trained carry her message of rehabilitation to hospitalized patients and to those patients who had left the hospital some time ago without ever receiving assistance.

By 1969, the potential of this rehabilitation endeavor became clear to the officers of the American Cancer Society, and we merged with the Reach to Recovery Program. The Society was able to offer its nationwide organizational structure of 58 divisions, 3,000 units and more than two million volunteers. We could help Terese Lasser build further on the solid foundation she had laid. Our interests were the same—*the welfare of the patient.* We needed her continuing leadership as the National Consultant to the Reach to Recovery Program. Her program would now benefit by medical supervision at the local level, the facilities of the American Cancer Society and the development of a team effort which included physician, nurse, physiotherapist and the trained Reach to Recovery Volunteer. The far-reaching results of this merger can be found in the Epilogue written by Dr. William M. Markel, Vice President for Service and Rehabilitation of the American Cancer Society.

The merger, or marriage, if you will, has been better than most. Terese Lasser serves as our inspiration for the concept of total rehabilitation of the mastectomy patient and as a regular 24-hour-a-day laborer for her dream of 1952. She brims with new ideas, new approaches and new devices, all designed to make a better life for women who have lost a breast.

It we had one complaint about the marriage, it would be this—Terese Lasser puts us to shame with her constant enthusiasm, tireless energy and abounding optimism. She is a rare woman indeed.

—Arthur I. Holleb, M.D.
Senior Vice President for Medical
Affairs and Research
American Cancer Society

I

Awakening

MORNING.

Or might it be evening?

Time matters so little, has so little meaning, that it really makes no difference . . .

You are alive!

Yes, but—?

How slowly you waken, on this day that will be unlike any other day in your life. A bell-note is sounding, a monotone, faintly, one-two-three-pause-one. Insistent, one-two-three-pause-one. Your mouth has never been so dry, or your eyelids so heavy. A numbness at the back of your head spreads down through your body . . . not a bad sensation—not good, either, but not bad. The air is weighted with a sweetly sterile smell. A white blob hovers, vanishes, returns, drifts away. From somewhere nearby there is the droning hum of bees in clover, then the bell-note sounds again—a different cadence? Yes: One-two-pause-one . . . unimportant. A small goldfish bowl floats up near the ceiling, and it seems to you in no way remarkable that a fishbowl should be up there suspended over your head.

One-two-pause-one. One-two-pause—

Memory is stirring.

The early years of your marriage: Wasn't there a sort of perennial joke in your family?—something about you "slaving" over a hot stove, unappreciated and unsung and yearning to "get away from it all"? Yes—"I know, I'll just check into the hospital for a week. To think of it! Seven lovely days with nothing to do but rest! And be waited on! And have breakfast served in bed every morning!"—to which your husband's reply had been something like, "Go to it. Don't worry about a thing here. I only hope the house will still be in one piece when you get home." As jokes go, hardly hilarious, to be sure, but the notion of your leaving them on their own for an entire day, let alone a week, was absurd enough to seem very funny at the time.

But now, somehow, it has happened.

Because this bed, surely, is a hospital bed? And that sweetish smell is surely the cloying aroma of a hospital? The white blob sliding in and out of focus must be—of course—a nurse; and that bell-note sounding again, one-pause-one-two, that would be an autocall summoning someone, and that fishbowl floating up near the ceiling is turning out to be no fishbowl at all but a bottle hanging from a metal rod, drip-dripping liquid into a tube that curves downward and disappears beneath your bedcovers.

You are coming wider awake, straining to order your confused thoughts.

You are in a hospital, no question about it, and that droning hum of bees in clover is a murmur of voices from across the room, the nurse talking with a scrubbed-looking stranger.

Wait, though.

Stranger? Don't you know that man?

Of course. He is the surgeon, the man your own doctor

sent you to see after a routine examination had discovered the lump in your breast.

Your reaction to that discovery, there in your doctor's office, had been stunned disbelief. You had been feeling so perfectly well, no aches or twinges anywhere, nothing that might have prepared you physically or psychologically for such a thing. A lump in your breast? But that was impossible, it could not be, it was something that happens to other women, one hears of it happening, and one is sympathetic and thankful not to be in their shoes, and then one puts it resolutely out of her mind. It might be that you have taken good health too much for granted, but you have at least always taken sensible care of your body, been reasonably faithful to a schedule of periodic checkups—

Nevertheless.

There had been a lump.

Your doctor is no alarmist. He had been calmly optimistic. "No cause for panic. None whatsoever. But let's be certain, shall we?"

So it had been arranged for you to see that man who is talking now to the nurse across the room. "A good man," your doctor had said, "one of the best." And to your enormous relief he, too, following his own examination, was reassuring.

But then, quite casually, he had added that he would have to perform a biopsy.

That had brought a chill. Was a biopsy an absolute must?

It was, indeed. The surgeon was very firm about taking out the lump and getting an immediate pathology report. He had added that the great majority of breast tumors are benign.

But suppose this one was not?

Cancer . . .

Dreaded, dreadful word, spoken in whispers when you were growing up, and seldom even whispered, then, in your hearing. In your adolescent mind it had taken on the aspect of a stigma, something tainted with shame, sinister, and in some mysterious way degrading. Grown women feared it, you knew that at a very early age, and somebody—a grandmother, or a great-aunt, or a second cousin, anyhow, somebody related—had it; you knew that, too, because mention of that person's name always brought a sad shaking of heads and a pity-filled pause in conversation.

Cancer!

Hearing the word applied to yourself that afternoon, even with such clinical detachment, had started all those old half-forgotten dreads jangling. Your doctor's "Only a few days in the hospital" and his "No cause for panic, the odds are all in your favor," intended to reassure, had not. Your initial disbelief gave way to an apprehension which grew steadily until the moment you checked into the hospital (when? Yesterday? Why has time become so elusive, so confused?). Once there, in an atmosphere of hushed efficiency and matter-of-fact expertise, your apprehension had lost some of its edge and your hands some of their clammy chill. And it was not long before you drifted off into a haze of indifference to pathology reports and everything else.

But you are coming out of that haze now, fast.

What did the biopsy show?

The report will be good, of course—unthinkable that it should be otherwise. What is the word again? Negative? Benign? Whatever, you want to hear it from that man across the room, the surgeon himself. And he seems on the verge of leaving. You would call out to him, but your mouth is too dry to manage more than an inaudible squeak. He is scribbling something—in your chart?—and does not look up for you to catch his eye. The nurse is intent on what the surgeon is saying, and she does not look up, either.

Shift your position in bed, that's it, do that and the movement may get their attention—

Pain lances through the numbness that is your body. To move your arm, one of your arms, is agony—but you can move the other, and you do move it. Your hand touches your side. For the first time you are aware of the bandage.

Bandage?

From midriff to neck, tight-wrapped as a mummy, you are bound in surgical gauze.

Somewhere deep inside you a switch is thrown and your mind goes blank. You do not want to think, you do not want to guess, you do not want to know. But in that moment you do know.

The impossible, the unthinkable, has happened.

Your breast has been removed.

When what has happened to you happened to me, some years ago, I could not even grope for answers to the dreadful questions forming in my mind. I had never known anyone who had had a breast removed. That I, personally, could ever experience such a thing was simply inconceivable. My "life style" (if that catch phrase had been in use then) would have been described in one word: *activity.* While attending New York University I'd squeezed time from studies for volunteer work in several hospitals. Later, when I was in the uniform of the Red Cross, driving an ambulance and doing welfare work had left enough hours to spare for me to serve as one of that organization's official cartographers.

Having married at eighteen, being a wife and mother were around-the-clock jobs, yet I had also been my husband's amanuensis in the preparation of the initial edition of J. K. Lasser's best-selling tax book, *Your Income Tax.* Even relaxation was an activity: I loved dancing, I loved parties and entertaining at home. Swimming, at the beach or in a pool, was a favorite sport, and at our country club I held the women's golf championship. In short, I was living a very full and a very active life.

The one thing I most certainly did not have time for was being ill.

My reaction when my doctor told me he had detected a small lump in my breast was more annoyance than apprehension. Precaution seemed such a nuisance! I checked into the hospital expecting surgery so minor that I made no mention of it to my husband; having suffered two heart attacks, he must not be alarmed by what I was sure was merely inconvenient "female trouble." He thought I was playing in a golf tournament at the moment I was being wheeled into the operating room.

Even minor surgery is never a pleasant prospect, of course. It is likely that I was really more apprehensive than I had admitted to myself. At least I recall that, awakening after the operation, my first thought—like your own—was *I am alive!*

But when told that my right breast had been removed, I wanted to shrivel up and die. How could I face life, a scarred woman? How could I go on, forever unfit for work or play? How could I look in a mirror again, knowing what I must see there and hating it?—sensing the revulsion in others and enduring the pity behind their curious stares? How could such a life be worth living?

And—most tormenting thought of all—*what about my husband?*

He was devoted to me—I was as confident of his love as any woman ever is confident. *But after this, what?* Suppose, in spite of his love and his devotion, he should be repelled by me? He was very much a man, after all, and for a man—any man—is love for a woman ever truly separated from desire? Was it possible for a man to desire a woman who wasn't whole? Suppose all my husband could feel for me now, all he would ever be able to feel, was pity?—so that never again would he need me, or reach for me as a man reaches for a woman?

If that were to be so, better not to be alive at all. . . .

There is, indeed, a Valley of Despair, desolate, solitary, swept by anguish, darkened by confusion. I, too, have been there.

Fortunately, today you need not linger in that valley.

The first step out of it is *acceptance* of your situation.

And there is help at hand to make acceptance easier. A Reach to Recovery Volunteer of the American Cancer Society will, with your surgeon's approval, visit you in the hospital to bring you this help. (About these dedicated volunteers—who they are, what they do—more later. Much more!)

In every one of the fifty states, divisions of the American Cancer Society carry on the Society's program of research, education and service to the cancer patient. And in virtually all these divisions there is a rehabilitation program in effect to meet the psychological, physical and cosmetic needs of the mastectomy patient. (Cosmetic needs pertain to every aspect of external appearance.)

This is Reach to Recovery, now a far-reaching program of a great voluntary health agency. Yet it grew out of my own needs and my own efforts so naturally and spontaneously that I am amazed, looking back, at what great strides have been made in rehabilitation in less than two decades.

Back in 1952, during my own first frightening days and nights in the hospital, the outlook seemed bleakly hopeless. Overwhelmed by anxieties so acute and so bewildering that I all but drowned in them, my mind surged with questions—some very practical but with no practical answers forthcoming, some rather foolish but nevertheless terribly serious to me, and some so highly personal I could not even bring myself to put them into words. How I ached to talk to another woman who had had the same experience and come through it, and so could counsel, and reassure, and understand!

But no such woman was available.

When I was told to start exercising, "What sort of exercise?" I asked my surgeon, a brilliant specialist and a very busy man.

He said the nurse would show me.

"Exercise of any kind," the nurse suggested, "just so that you move your arm."

Exercise of any kind . . . no guidance, really. No actual supervision. No positive program of postoperative mental and physical therapy to make a woman's comeback to her former way of life a challenging project rather than an ordeal of trial and error, distress and heartache.

One question I did not ask myself: *Could* I come back to

my usual active life? That I refused to doubt even for a moment. Just try hard enough, I told myself, and you will improve. Trying meant holding fast to confidence about the future. It meant working out exercises that would give me full use of my affected arm. My enthusiasm for golf led me to try a golf swing as exercise, and a rubber ball I had used in the past, clutching and releasing it to strengthen my golf grip, became another helpful exercise. Of course I made the mistake of overdoing in my zeal to speed up my recovery. But on the whole I was encouraged, as I could see the progress I was making. I discovered what helped me most was reaching. I worked hard at devising new exercises that would force me to reach. In fact, when my own early volunteer efforts got organized and I was trying to think of a name for my work, I knew that "Reach" had to be part of the title.

But exercise was just part of what I had to reach for. I had to find out—sometimes by painful trial and error—how to cope with all the problems of dress and wardrobe adjustment that breast surgery makes us face. To begin with, I had to discover where to shop for an artificial breast form. I didn't even know they were called prostheses—or even how to pronounce the word (it's pross-*thees*-ease). Well, it wasn't easy, and I'm happy that things are better organized now. Today your Reach to Recovery Volunteer of your local ACS unit will provide you with a list of stores that specialize in prostheses and with other useful shopping information.

It wouldn't have occurred to me as I was slowly working away at solving my problems that I was taking the first step to helping other women solve theirs. But all journeys begin with a single step.

A few months after my surgery I heard that Helen V. B., with whom I'd once worked in the Red Cross, had just undergone this operation and was having an extremely bad time. She was so profoundly depressed that she refused to talk to anyone and would see no visitors.

A mutual friend suggested that I might be able to get through to this woman something of what I had been learning about recovery after a mastectomy, and perhaps give her morale a much needed boost.

I resisted the suggestion. It was so soon after my operation that I had not yet resolved all my own problems of recovery, either emotionally or physically. It was one thing to have confidence in the future for myself; it would be something else to instill confidence in someone else. Helen V. B. was not a close friend; there was no reason she should want to see me, or trust me, or listen to anything I had to say. In her place, wouldn't I consider such personal advice from a casual acquaintance a gratuitous intrusion upon privacy? In her place wouldn't I . . . ?

But I had been in her place—and had longed to talk with another woman who had shared the same experience, who could advise, and reassure, and above all understand. Might not what had been true for me also be true for this woman? Did her refusal to talk to anyone mean she would not talk to another woman who had had a mastectomy? Did her refusal to see any visitors mean she would not see someone who, hopefully, might be a bit more than just a visitor?

I telephoned the hospital and spoke to Helen V. B.'s nurse, who listened to my request to come and talk to her patient. But when she relayed my request, the answer was no, Mrs. V. B. did not want to see me. On the chance that she might change her mind, I left my phone number with the nurse and hung up.

My feelings were mixed: part disappointment, part relief.

I had not really felt ready for the challenge of getting through to a woman plunged in the depths of grief and despondency. And yet there was just a chance that I might have gotten through, and been able to help her. Denied that chance, I suddenly wanted it very much.

Early the next morning the same nurse called to say that Mrs. V. B.'s doctor, learning of my call, had urged Helen to change her mind about seeing me—the doctor, too, felt it might relieve his patient's depression to talk with another woman who had had a mastectomy and was recovering from it. The nurse had been instructed to say I could visit Helen that afternoon.

So now the question was, How to make the most of this opportunity? A thought flashed through my mind: *One picture is worth a thousand words.* To provide Helen with visual proof that my appearance was unchanged, that I had the full use of my arm so soon after my operation, would be better for her morale than a thousand words of encouragement.

When I walked into the hospital room a few hours later, I was wearing a formfitting knit dress, makeup very carefully applied, and a hat borrowed from a friend. Hats are anathema to me, I never wear one if I can avoid it, and I owned none suitable for my ensemble that afternoon. The reason one had been borrowed for this occasion was that when we had worked for the Red Cross, Helen was always amused when I snatched off my uniform hat the moment we were out of sight of headquarters; the same impetuous gesture now might reestablish an old rapport as well as demonstrate that loss of mobility in an affected arm need be merely temporary.

Well, the snatching off of the hat produced no flicker of amusement, no sign of rapport old or new. When the nurse left us alone, the woman in bed looked at me without, apparently, any recognition whatsoever. When I spoke she did not reply. The dark eyes stared, unblinking, clouded with pain and resentment. I wanted to back away, to apologize for having come, to escape from the weight of that silent suffering.

Then I remembered my own feelings, lying in just such a bed. Instead of backing away, I drew up a chair and sat down and began to talk quietly, almost at random, concerned less for the words than for the thought behind them—that it's possible for a woman to discover within herself wellsprings of strength that she did not know she possessed, tenderness and perception far beyond anything she has ever known before. Rather than being less a person after this operation, I said, a woman's femininity can be enhanced, her ability to love increased, her awareness of her womanhood heightened. I said I was finding all this to be true, myself.

And from Helen V. B.—no response. No movement. No sound. Nothing even to indicate she had been listening.

I stood up.

"I'm running late, Helen," I said briskly, "and I've been on the go since seven this morning." Slowly her head turned on the pillow. I went on, "A regular merry-go-round! Eighteen holes of golf, then a quick swim, and you know what it was driving in here fighting that traffic." At long last, a reaction—her eyes were widening in a kind of entranced disbelief. "I'd stay longer," I added, raising both arms to put on the hat again, "but I really must get home to change for a cocktail party."

She spoke then, in a choked whisper. "You haven't gone through what I have. They didn't do to you what they've done to me."

"Yes," I said, "yes, my dear, they did," and I leaned over, gently took her hand and held it to my left breast, then to my right. "One is mine, Helen. Can you tell which is which?"

I stepped back and waited.

She started to speak, and could not. Her eyes filled with tears. She shook her head, but she understood. She knew she was not alone. Color came into her face, and a glowing into her eyes that could only be hope coming alive. She motioned for my hand, and pressed it against her cheek.

At that precise moment, I think, the idea for Reach to Recovery was born.

II

You and the Man in Your Life

IT IS A SOBERING FACT that of every hundred women in these United States, six will some day develop breast cancer.

It is the leading cancer in incidence and mortality among women today, according to statistics issued by the American Cancer Society. An estimated 71,000 new cases will be diagnosed in 1972, and according to a spokesman for the ACS, "It is the most costly in terms of medical bills."

But 1,500,000 Americans have been *cured of cancer,* and of these almost 250,000 have had mastectomies—a quarter-million of us, alive and well, each the same person we were before the operation, with the potential of becoming a better wife, a better mother, a better woman in every sense of the word.

The ACS reports very real progress in the management of breast cancer. Early detection, accurate diagnosis and prompt treatment have made the rate of cure as high as 85 percent today. With confidence spurred by this and by other progress made during the past decade, the ACS entered the seventies resolved to make it the decade which would see a decisive step toward complete control of all types of cancer. And as its programs of research and education advanced upon that objective, the Society's program of service to the patient was being expanded beyond the most optimistic dreams of only a few short years ago.

When I told my surgeon about my idea for Reach to Recovery, he thought it over very carefully before he expressed an opinion. I was visiting his office daily at the time, following my own surgery, and he had been obliged to listen daily to my indignation about the lack of guidance for post-mastectomy patients. Finally, "Do something about it," he had told me, and now that I had an idea of what that "something" should be, his approval of it was very important.

He said he did approve—but with a word of caution. "You know the old saw about new ideas, Lassie."

If I'd ever known it, I'd forgotten it.

" 'Every new idea,' " the doctor said, " 'has something of the pain and peril of childbirth.' " He added, "Anyone who has ever tried to promote a new idea will tell you how true that is."

Was he telling me there would be problems in transforming Reach to Recovery from an idea into reality? I expected that. I was also confident that I could handle the problems.

He nodded. "Just so you're not counting on clear sledding with nary a bump along the way. Some surgeons will approve, as I do. Some will not. There'll be those who'll say that postoperative rehabilitation should be provided only by professionals, not lay people like yourself, Lassie." He scribbled a name on a slip of paper and handed it to me. "Do you know this woman?"

The name was not familiar.

"Perhaps you can help her," the doctor said. "I'll tell her nurse I've asked you to look in this afternoon." He rose and held out his hand. "Get going on your idea," he said, "and good luck."

So, for the second time within a week I was walking into a hospital room wearing a carefully chosen formfitting dress (this one with a colorful scarf attached), makeup carefully applied, and a hat.

The room faced west, and the afternoon sun was streaming in. The shade on the window was lowered halfway. It occurred to me that if I could coax that shade to snap up and whip around its roller, then reach up to lower it, an impression would be made on the patient far in excess of simply reaching up to remove my hat.

Squinting toward the window, I remarked that the sun was in my eyes—might the shade be lowered? The patient nodded indifferently. I went to the window, praying that the ratchet stops on the roller would slip. And obligingly they did so. The shade shot up, banging against the top of the window. I tch-tched, got up onto a chair, reached with my left hand to the left corner of the shade and with my right hand to the right corner, and tugged until it unrolled and came down to stop where I wanted it.

Stepping down off the chair, I saw the patient staring at me thoughtfully. "You can use both arms, can't you?"

"Of course. Can't you?"

"I can use my arms, but—" She hesitated. Then she said, "I have trouble walking."

This was not at all what I had expected. Had something happened to her feet, or her legs?

"No." With an effort, she sat up. "If you'll help me off the bed, I'll show you what I mean."

Together we got her up onto her feet. Her problem became obvious: A heavy, pendulous-breasted woman, when she stood erect and the remaining breast was unsupported, she was unbalanced, with a posture so awkward and a feeling of being so lopsided that it was difficult for her to maintain her equilibrium.

The solution which we devised was both simple and effective—a kerchief-sling support for her remaining breast, which restored her balance as well as her self-confidence.

Should you, too, experience an off-balance feeling after your operation, here is how to make such a sling: Request a piece of soft material about 40 inches square and fold it to form a triangle. Ask your nurse to help you fit your breast into what is about to become a cup-support for its weight. Bring the tip of the triangle upward; bring one end around in back and down over your shoulder, to meet the other end in front. Do not tie a knot where it may cause pressure upon your shoulder. Instead, make a small pad (a 4 x 4-inch pad or any soft fabric will do nicely), place it beneath the folded-under ends of the sling, and pin securely together. Usually this is most comfortably arranged on the collarbone area. Support is assured by nipping the sling material beneath your breast so that it forms a cup shape in the lower edge toward your arm, then fastening it with a safety pin to hold that shape. Another pin is used in the same way on top of the cup.

Those first walks following your operation may frequently be made more comfortable if you use an underarm rest on which to prop your affected hand for support.

Put together with your surgeon's approval and your nurse's help, this "rest" is a cylinderlike roll 6 to 8 inches in diameter and about 18 inches in length, which you place under your armpit as close and as high as is comfortable. It may be made of twelve small or six large hospital pads ("chux"), or any cushiony material that you can depend on not to sag.

Tie the roll tightly in three places: the middle, and 5

inches in from either end. Cover the roll with some plastic material and then with a soft towel or a pillowcase. To each of the end ties of the roll attach a 27-inch length of 2-inch bandage; allow these ends to dangle loose for a moment. Position the roll under your armpit as high as possible. When it is comfortable there, your nurse can bring the two dangling ends of 2-inch bandage together over the opposite shoulder, place a soft pad beneath ends of bandage where knot will come and tie them securely.

Simply by resting your hand and arm on this roll during your walks, you will find your comfort much increased.

After that visit to his patient, my doctor sent me to see several others during the weeks that followed.

What was helpful for one woman was not necessarily helpful for another, but a universality of suffering surely did exist—the same tormenting questions crying for answers, the same fears begging to be quieted, the same sense of loss of womanhood needing to be contradicted.

Following radical breast surgery, those women were like wounded soldiers returning from battle, frantically seeking guidance from someone, somewhere, in order to adjust to life. I talked about this with my doctor. I listened carefully to what he had to say, I talked and listened to other doctors and to nurses, and of course to the patients themselves. I rethought my own ideas, and tried to improve them. And out of all this the rehabilitation program that was to become Reach to Recovery began to acquire definite shape and substance—almost, quite literally, a vibrant life of its own.

But my doctor had been right that a new idea does indeed have something of the pain and peril of childbirth!

It was painful, for instance, to discover that I was sometimes suspected of being motivated by personal gain; more than once, a cynical "What's in all this for you?" rocked me back on my heels. It was painful to find that professionals who recognized the desperate need for postoperative rehabilitation were sometimes uncooperative simply because I lacked formal training as a therapist. Most painful, most disheartening of all, was encountering opposition to this new idea just because it *was* new.

Of course, pain and peril notwithstanding, childbirth does go on and a child does get itself born.

So it was with Reach to Recovery.

Disappointment was balanced by encouragement: my doctor felt strongly that the time had come for something like this to be done. Many other doctors, and many nurses, agreed. Those first patients had been visibly helped—physically, psychologically and cosmetically. And my husband's faith in the idea and in my ability to carry it out never wavered.

The program's core was my own experience in achieving maximum mental and emotional recovery as well as physical health after having a breast removed. This is what enabled me to speak to other women in the same situation with understanding, hope and confidence. As a kind of practical "How to" guide for these women, I decided to put this experience on paper and the first *Reach to Recovery Manual* went into the typewriter. My husband offered to finance the publication of ten thousand copies, to be distributed without charge to mastectomy patients whose surgeons approved of their receiving one.

When the *Manual* was in galley form, an opportunity came to test its impact upon a man whose acceptance or rejection would be a major clue to the future of Reach to Recovery.

The man was Dr. O'M., a distinguished surgeon in Seattle, and he was to be the first doctor to see what I had written. My husband had been invited to speak at the University of Washington, and I persuaded him to take me—and my *Manual*—along for company. Our hosts out there set up an appointment for me to meet with Dr. O'M.

While I read aloud from the galley, the doctor listened impassively. Fingertips pressed together, eyes lidded, his manner was patient and courteous—and, as far as I could tell, totally unimpressed. My heart sank. I read on to the end, and looked up.

He had swiveled around to gaze pensively out the window. His thoughts, surely, were a million miles away. More than likely he had forgotten my presence altogether.

If ever there was a longer, more aching moment of silence, I have never lived through it.

Then, abruptly, he swiveled to face me. And he was nodding emphatically.

"Good!" Dr. O'M. said. "How soon can you supply us with five hundred copies?"

Of course I was overjoyed. It was the beginning of a flood of requests for my little yellow *Manual* (I have never wanted to change the cheerful sunny color, though the 1969 revised edition is now the 14th printing). My husband generously let us use his office for storing and shipping the *Manual.* Thanks to his patience and the help of his wonderful secretary, Katherine Maddrey, his business did not suffer too much with the addition of a one-woman publishing program. And all that it entailed.

Important as was my husband's role in getting the Reach to Recovery Program started, more important by far was his role as the man in my life during those days and nights immediately following my operation.

His patience and understanding were tried as never before. It was not easy for either of us, and it did not happen in a week or a month, but together we did work our way through that critical period so that I emerged from it reassured of his love, knowing my fears about his pitying me had been groundless, feeling needed and wanted, desirable and desired.

For a woman, this renewed confidence in herself is the most precious of all gifts. 1647040

And only the man in her life can give it to her.

We are all of us so incomplete in ourselves! That is life's riddle to which nature's answer is the sexual relationship. When that relationship works, you complete your husband as a man and he completes you as a woman. Life, then, can be a very good thing. But when the relationship fails, the joy of loving fails, and life can drain into a shell of emptiness.

Because of the surgery you have had, that shell of emptiness looms agonizingly close. It did for me, just after my operation. It does for most women at such a time. So it is important, now, more than ever before, to be sure that you truly do understand fully your own role in the sexual relationship. A woman may fail to achieve the joy of loving because her comprehension of her role in it falls short of what, in fact, that role is.

Recently I received a letter from a young woman in Texas who had undergone a mastectomy only a short time ago. She described herself as being twenty-five, the mother of two little girls, and went on, "My worst moments were dressing in the morning and undressing in the evening. Luckily, my husband was willing to share these moments." (They should be shared, by all means. The husband who leaves the room when his wife is dressing or undressing makes a grave mistake—far from her thinking it is considerate of him, she will be convinced of what she already dreads, that he cannot bear to look at her.) "The hardest thing for me to accept," the letter continued, "was that my husband, who is only twenty-four years old, has to live with me like this forever. But I've accepted it, because he has. He's mature for his years and a wonderful guy. He says he really doesn't mind the scar at all. What he tells me is, 'I'm a leg man, myself.' Between you and me, I'm making sure that he is reminded mine are as good as ever!"

Clearly, this couple's sexual problems were minimal after this operation. The husband was being understanding; both had kept a sense of humor; and—most important—the wife was still proud of her femininity. A personal affirmation of femininity is particularly essential following this surgery. *It is through a demonstrated pride in her own female nature that a woman shapes the quality of the sexual relationship in her marriage*—psychologists tell us this is so, and our own marriages, when we stop to think of this aspect of them, prove it is, indeed, a fact.

And it remains no less true for you, now, than it is for women who have not had this surgery.

Your doctor may have said to you, as mine did to me, "You are every bit the person you always were. The operation has in no way changed what you were, the essential You"—meaning that the intangible uniqueness which is your psyche, your spiritual being, has not been excised by the surgeon's knife. Also that the rapport you have had with your man—whatever compatibility of temperament, tastes and intellect you enjoy together—is beyond the reach of scalpel and suture.

It is good to know that the essential You is intact.

But what worries a woman is, when has any man ever been stirred to physical passion by her psyche? When has a husband's sexual desire been aroused by those intangible attributes of his wife's which cannot be seen, touched, or caressed?

The answer is, *Never!* . . . isn't it? Or is it?

Beware the error of underestimating your man.

There was a time when women believed that sex for a man was solely a matter of externals, of surface sensations rather than spiritual sensitivity—his ardor aroused by sight and scent stimuli, his erotic pleasure an entirely physical response on an entirely physical plane. That was also the time when it was believed that all women possessed an inborn understanding of the male psychology, whereas no man was able to probe the feminine mystique. Echoes of that illusion persist in the notion that the male animal fails grossly in sensitivity and perception—that as the only one of God's creatures to "eat when he is not hungry, drink when he is not thirsty, and make love at all seasons" he may be summed up as part foolish sinner and part exasperating angel, a simple being whose appetites are materialistic and whose satisfactions are self-centered—all in all, hardly reassuring to one who must depend on him, as you must now, for the ultimate in patience and understanding.

The sensible woman, however, will take the male animal not for what he is said to be, or ought to be, but rather for what he is.

For example, this man of yours: During the crises, major and minor, of your marriage, all the days and nights and months and years of your life together, surely he has proven himself something more than a simple brew of sexual appetite and spiritual calluses?

Think back, say, to your early courtship.

You may not have been aware at the time that the person with whom this man of yours fell in love was not actually you, that is to say, your physical self, so much as it was his own romantic idealizing of you. Psychologists tell us that this is characteristic of the male animal during his courtship period: sexual desire and physical passion play muted second fiddles to a theme of cerebral adoration. It is even unlikely that your measurements, so-called, had much to do with his initial attraction to you; more probably he was drawn by the shape of your mouth, your smile or the sound of your laugh, the color of your eyes, or your hair, or simply the way you moved—reliable surveys report that many men consider that a woman's buttocks are her most attractive feature. Whatever it was that caught his eye, his imagination then went to work spinning daydreams which left you—the real you—waiting in the wings for a cue before making an entrance into his life. When he whispered, "I'm in love with you!" he meant he was in love with a vision fashioned from his secret longings, a mental image which you might scarcely have recognized as yourself but which he set upon a pedestal and lighted with an aura of dreamy worship.

The point is (and do bear this in mind as you prepare to face the future) the man in your life is quite sensitive enough, and perceptive enough, to respond to your womanhood now as he did before—*provided you yourself rise to the challenge of that womanhood, now.*

Some time ago I met with a woman in her thirties, personable and attractive, but obviously very distressed. Her home was in the Midwest, her husband was an obstetrician, and several months prior to coming to my home late one afternoon she had undergone a mastectomy.

The reason for her distress was that since her operation her husband had not resumed sexual relations.

When I asked whether she had discussed this with him, she shook her head. It was, she insisted, up to him to take the initiative, and because he had not, a breach between them was widening into a real estrangement.

Treading carefully, I suggested that it was possible, in his anxiety to do what was right and best for her, he had been waiting for some sign that his advances would be welcomed. I pointed out that very often a husband's emotional adjustment to this situation is as dependent upon his wife's attitude as her own adjustment is dependent upon his.

In our scheme of things, marriage is a climate in which a man's courtship whisper, "I'm in love with you!" deepens to "I love you." The difference is notable; it pivots on his wish to nourish and protect, to act for the happiness of someone other than himself. His near-ecstatic worship of a dream-idol comes down to earth, within the framework of marriage, to become everyday thoughtfulness and affection for a person outside himself—his wife. The spur to this transformation, of course, is that intimacy of body and emotion we call the sexual relationship—which is at its best only when erotic response is mutual.

Had this troubled woman enjoyed a good sexual relationship with her husband before her operation? Yes, she had. Did she feel now, since the operation, able to bring to that relationship all that she had before? Well, hardly. Did that mean that she felt herself to be less a woman now?—because if so, was it surprising if her husband's sexual response to her was also less?

We talked a long time that afternoon. When she left it was growing dark, but she took away with her the light of one of the most enduring of all verities: *The better the sexual relationship is in a marriage, the less it depends upon the purely physical qualities of either partner.*

She promised to let me know if her marriage came together again. We worked out a little code: If all went well, she would send me a postcard saying simply that her garden was in bloom, and I would understand.

But how sad that there had already been such heartache—and how unnecessary. Because, fundamentally, it is a woman's own attitude that determines the quality of marital sex. If, prior to a mastectomy, that relationship was based upon mutual love and desire, and was good and satisfying, it will be good and satisfying afterward unless the woman's own attitude decrees otherwise.

You yourself, for instance, have doubtless discovered that passive consent to the act of love on your part seldom provides real joy for your husband. True, he is the active aggressor, but it is you who evoke and guide that aggression. Passivity or unresponsiveness on your part is an almost insurmountable barrier to consummation for him.

All along, in the act of love, it has been your feminine attitude which has been primarily in control. All along, it was your resourcefulness in expressions of love-enjoyment that sustained your husband's sexual ardor.

In short, it has always been your demonstrated pride in your womanhood which has determined—*and can continue to determine*—the quality of the sexual relationship in your marriage. Nothing that has happened is a reason for you to be any less proud of your womanhood now. Nothing has lessened your ability to love, or diminished your innate femininity. Your spirit and your intellect are intact. And your capacity for tenderness and understanding may well be greater than ever before.

My friend from the Midwest found this to be so. Three weeks after her visit a card arrived bearing the postmark of her home town. It contained ten beautiful words: "My garden is in full bloom. Thank you, thank you."

Even before that first *Reach to Recovery Manual* came off the press, it was clear that the need for a program of postoperative rehabilitation was greater than I had supposed.

Overnight, it seemed, my correspondence doubled, tripled, quadrupled—letters from women who had heard what I was trying to do and sought advice about exercises, or information on bras and clothing and prostheses, or simply wanted to help—and every letter calling for a personal reply. I began scouring department stores and specialty shops for the latest and best prostheses, and bathing suits, and grooming aids to which women who inquired could be referred. My shopping trips became safaris of exploration. Visits to hospitals were stepped up. I continued to call on patients whenever permitted to do so; I talked to doctors, singly and in groups; I talked with social workers and physiotherapists; I asked and obtained permission to speak to graduating classes of nurses, because it was the nurse who would be the logical emissary for the Reach to Recovery Program: Being a woman herself, she would have an instinctive comprehension of a mastectomy patient's emotions, and she was the one who would have the most intimate and continuous contact with the patient during those dark hours immediately following surgery.

All of this, needless to say, had a certain impact on my private life.

Our social activities were sharply curtailed. A vacation trip with friends was twice postponed, then canceled altogether. Our cleaning woman muttered unhappily about not being allowed to move my typewriter or "neaten up" the drop-leaf table I had pressed into service as a desk. Our daughter, away at school, wrote that it was impossible to reach us by phone because the line was even busier than when she had been at home tying it up for hours. Our son suggested a separate phone for Reach to Recovery, with a separate listing in the directory. My husband, whose own work schedule always disregarded clocks entirely, suggested dryly that I try to schedule one evening a week, uninterrupted, to brief him on what was going on.

And yet truly no one, family or friends—even our cleaning woman—was anything less than encouraging, enthusiastic, and keenly interested in the project.

As a matter of fact, it was the cleaning woman who brought Rachel S. to see me.

Here was a problem, in the person of Rachel, to which I'd given no thought until that moment: the problem of the unmarried woman who, faced with a mastectomy, is beset by doubts about her personal appeal and marital prospects following a mastectomy.

Rachel was in her twenties, lived alone, and worked as a ticket seller in a neighborhood movie house. She had had two cysts removed from her breast; now she had discovered another lump and lived in terror over the possibility of eventually having to undergo a mastectomy. She had discussed this with a friend who had had "that operation" a year before. The friend told Rachel that as a result of this surgery she, the friend, could no longer become pregnant. Poor Rachel was sure that not only would a mastectomy cost her a chance at matrimony, but, should some man ever wish to marry her, she would be unable to bear him a child.

How tragic the misery that a single grain of misunderstanding can cause!

Because Rachel had indeed misunderstood her friend.

After urging her to have a frank talk with her doctor, which Rachel was too frightened to do (again, how tragic!), I questioned her about this friend—who turned out to be much older than Rachel, married, and the mother of five children. In addition to postoperative radiation therapy, she had also had X-ray treatments on her abdomen (to her ovaries) so that she would stop menstruating and simultaneously become infertile.

Apparently more was involved in Rachel's friend's case than just the removal of a breast. I pointed this out to Rachel, again urged her to see her doctor without delay, and assured her that some women—after gaining their surgeon's approval for the pregnancy—do bear children after a mastectomy.

As to whether such surgery would lessen Rachel's marital prospects, several of the letters then on my desk said, in effect, "No!": "I married after my operation and have a very fine understanding husband"; "We met six months after my operation and have just come back from a wonderful honeymoon"; "This dear man does not consider me damaged in any sense of the word, so we've set the date. . . ." These excerpts I read aloud, hoping to ease Rachel's mind a little on this score.

Had today's computer analyses of marriage patterns among young people been in vogue then, they would have offered even more encouragement.

A recent sampling of students by a computer-dating service

has revealed that college men, in weighing what they admire most in femininity, rated friendliness and honesty on a par with physical attractiveness (see Vance Packard's *The Sexual Wilderness*). Undeniably, the female breast is erotically appealing to these young males—any poll's subjects must be products of their culture, and we have in today's America what is probably the most breast-oriented culture in the world. Nevertheless, few men make the decision to marry because they are spellbound by breasts. One highly regarded study found that what really quickens the pace of courtship today is when a couple shares *ideals* about personal goals in life and *ideas* about who is to do what in the marriage—it is this sort of compatibility which, according to Packard's in-depth report, most often brings a young woman and a young man together at the altar.

And we have it on the word of this same authority that nine out of ten people entering their twenties will be married before they are thirty; these are odds that favor young women like Rachel—mastectomy notwithstanding—having at least a chance at matrimony.

As for Rachel herself, a short while after her visit she went back to the city in North Carolina where her parents lived. There, in the words of our cleaning woman, "The doctor who brought her into the world" examined her and sent her to a surgeon; it was decided that a mastectomy was necessary, Rachel had had it and was "doing just fine."

Several months later, a clipping arrived in the mail. It was one of those fine-print, back-page columns of vital statistics, *Marriage License Applied For.* And circled in red was Rachel's name. That was all, but it was enough.

In the years since, I hope she has never forgotten that all-important key to marital happiness for all of us who have had a mastectomy: *You are the same person you were before the operation—and can become even better!*

You yourself, I hope, will always remember this. How you think of yourself is how the man in your life will think of you. *Unless you make the mistake of feeling inferior, he will not think of you as being inferior.* Remember that his sexual response to you has always depended basically upon your own pride in your femininity and your boundless capacity, as a woman, for love and devotion. Womanly pride . . . a capacity for love . . .

Nurture that capacity and that pride—you still possess both, provided you do nurture them—and the man in your life will be the loving and devoted companion you need to help you over the hurdles that lie ahead.

III

Reach—and Reach Again

FROM THE VERY OUTSET, Reach to Recovery's heart (in the warmest sense of the word) has been its woman-to-woman aspect—one woman who has been through it all talking straightforwardly to any other woman who is just starting on her road to recovery.

This was my goal when I started the program in 1953, and it is still the prime objective of Reach to Recovery now that it has been coordinated into the Service and Rehabilitation program of the American Cancer Society. The merger took place in 1969. As National Reach to Recovery Consultant and Coordinator, I am gratified that our Volunteers can now help more patients and doctors than ever before without in any way interfering with the doctor-patient relationship.

When your doctor approves a visit from a well-trained Reach to Recovery Volunteer, he does so in the confidence that your morale will be lifted, that the Volunteer will explain and demonstrate the proper exercises, and that she will urge you to accept the realities of your situation—*such acceptance is the first positive step toward renewed good health.*

The Volunteer also brings, as a gift, a *Reach to Recovery* Kit. These kits consist of a temporary breast form which, pinned inside your nightgown, is an immediate boost to morale; a rubber ball on an elastic string and a special plastic-coated rope, both basic equipment for the exercises which, provided your doctor gives his permission, should begin in the hospital; a copy of the *Manual;* a reference list of sources for prostheses and grooming aids; other brochures; and, if you are married, an important message for your husband. (I'll be discussing all this in detail as we go along.)

You will be shown how to squeeze and relax the rubber ball to strengthen your hand; how to throw the ball on its elastic string and catch it on the rebound, to strengthen your arm and shoulder muscles; how to toss the plastic-coated rope up over the top of a door to make a pulley of it for raising and lowering your affected arm. The Volunteer will explain that doing these exercises may cause some pain at first, but that this will lessen and soon disappear. Then she will suggest that you take deep breaths, relax . . . and then continue, because although you must not get overtired, neither should you coddle yourself when it comes to exercising.

She may talk with you about courage, and the fact that you are the same person you were before your operation—and can be even more of a woman now; that you are not alone, that many women have felt their inner security and sense of self threatened, as you do now, and have been restored to a glowing, enriched life—as you, too, can be.

The American Cancer Society has been careful to include only doctor-approved exercises in its Reach to Recovery Program. Because your surgeon alone is qualified to inform you on the details of your surgery (remember, there are different ways a mastectomy may be performed), it is vital that you follow his instructions to the letter—when to start, how far to go, when to stop.

All Reach to Recovery exercises have one basic principle—*reach!* For instance:

REACH!—TO YOUR HAIR

Hair-brushing exercise

Sit at a night table, or where you can prop your elbow to support your affected arm. Take brush in hand and raise it slowly to your hair. Don't bend your head to meet it—keep your head up, your shoulders even. Limit brushing at first to that side of your head nearest the brush.

Gradually work around to the other side, reaching further, little by little, until you are able to brush the entire head. Do not overdo. Rest when you feel you must—but keep at it! Persistence rewards you by hastening your recovery, and the appearance of your hair will be improved in the bargain.

And again, for instance:

REACH!—TO CRUMPLE PAPER

Paper-crumpling exercise

Still seated, with your forearm resting on the table, have a pile of flat sheets of old newspapers (each sheet about 11″ x 15″) placed so that your hand just touches one corner of them.

Sheet by sheet, one at a time, draw the paper into your hand and slowly crumple it into a ball. Then discard it. By reaching to get the paper, then reaching to discard it, you will begin to strengthen the muscles of your forearm and hand.

In doing other Reach to Recovery exercises, posture is most important: Stand erect, head up, arms at your sides. Assure proper balance by placing your feet hip-width apart with the balls of the feet carrying your weight. Working in front of a mirror will help you to keep your shoulders even—this is essential. Work barefoot, or in low-heeled shoes. All exercises are—always—done slowly. Continue for only short periods at first.

And if it hurts, do not be dismayed. Exercises hurt most of us when we began them. If pain does occur, it does not usually last long if you are faithful in doing the exercises. Take deep breaths and relax. Do these exercises daily, day after day, and you will be delighted with your over-all improvement. You'll be surprised, too, at the speed with which untrained muscles can be trained to perform new tasks.

Remember, first check your posture. Then—

REACH!—FOR A RUBBER BALL

Rubber ball exercise

The kit which you were given in the hospital by a Volunteer contains a rubber ball attached to an elastic string. (Toy departments in most stores stock this item—you may recall it as a favorite toy of childhood.)

Place the ball in your palm. Tighten a grip on it. Squeeze. Relax. Repeat. And repeat. You should feel muscles responding all through your arm.

Next (keeping shoulders even, feet hip-width apart) throw the ball in any direction away from the body, and as the elastic snaps it back up, try to catch it. (It doesn't really matter if you don't.) Try to throw it from the shoulder, a little farther each time.

REACH!—TO CLIMB A WALL

Wall-climbing exercise

Face the wall with your forehead resting against it. Balance is especially important here, so be sure your posture is correct—

feet hip-width apart, shoulders even, arms at your side, weight on the balls of your feet.

Now slowly raise your arms to place your palms flat against the wall. Move your hands slowly upward against the wall. Keep reaching upward until you have brought both arms close to your ears, your *elbows straight,* and both hands as high as possible on the wall.

Lower your arms to shoulder height and start over. Do this several times a day.

With practice, your "climb" will increase. Mark your upward progress on the wall with a pencil or a piece of adhesive or Scotch tape. Each day try to reach beyond the mark of the previous day.

REACH!—WITH A PULLEY

Pulley exercise

If you have a Reach to Recovery Kit, use the plastic-coated rope that comes in it. Otherwise, secure a length of rope 5 feet long and knot it heavily at both ends. (Or fold a bandage into three lengths of 5 feet each, with large knots at both ends of the triple thickness, to make a "rope.") Put pencils or any smooth firm object through the knots to make the rope easier to hold.

If you are a slight person whose weight will not put too much pull on a shower rod, you can toss one end of the rope over the rod and seat yourself straddling the tub's edge. Or if it is more convenient, hang the rope over a sturdy hook on a door or a wall (distance of hook from the floor should be about 7 feet) and sit on a chair placed beneath the hook.

Take hold of the rope on your affected side first.

With the knots positioned firmly between the third and fourth fingers, pull downward with the arm opposite the site of the operation—which will raise the affected arm slowly upward.

Bring it on up until your hand is as close to your nose as possible, with elbows straight; then lower it slowly.

Do this Reach to Recovery pulley exercise five times in the morning and five times in the evening, at first. Increase this count gradually, a little more each day, until you're doing it about 25 times a day.

REACH!—WITH A JUMP ROPE

Jump-rope exercise

This rope should be about as long as you can spread your arms apart. Knot it at both ends. Fasten one end to a doorknob or a bureau-drawer pull; hold the other knotted end in your affected hand. Be sure that your elbow is slightly bent and the rope is slack between you and the door or the bureau.

Place your other hand on your hip, to help maintain your balance. Stand at right angles to the bureau or the door. Check posture—head up, shoulders even, arms at sides. Look straight ahead.

Now, without bending your waist, raise your affected arm out fairly straight, sideways, toward the bureau or door, and start swinging the rope from the shoulder in a clockwise direction. After five swings clockwise, reverse the direction and do the same number counterclockwise.

Move in closer to the door or bureau to make your circular swings wider. Each day, try to widen the circles, and gradually increase the number of swings from five in each direction to as many as you can manage without unduly tiring yourself.

REACH!—AND BEND ELBOWS

Shoulder exercise

(This is not suggested as a hospital exercise. It can be highly beneficial, however, to help relax neck tension when you go home.) Raise your left arm sideways up to shoulder height. Bend your elbow. Roll your shoulder in its socket as far back and around as possible. Do this clockwise five times, counterclockwise five times.

Repeat with your right arm.

Next, rotate both arms in this way simultaneously, around and around, back and back until your shoulder blades almost touch. This not only relieves back-neck tensions but it will help you meet such practical challenges as fastening a bra and zippering a dress up the back.

Do be persistent about exercising. You are, literally, reaching toward your maximum recovery by doing so. Do not, however, tire yourself or overdo. And if in the beginning you need help to do them, ask for help.

To give greater suppleness to your arm and shoulder on the side of the operation, these additional exercises may prove helpful—try them using your affected hand:

Facing a door, close your fingers loosely around the knob; maintaining this relaxed grip, slowly turn until your back is to the door.

Raise your hand diagonally across your body and place it firmly upon the opposite shoulder.

Bring your hand behind your body, bend your elbow and reach to grasp the opposite elbow.

There is no reason exercises need become a burden, and to avoid that happening, try varying the routine. Indulge in a change of pace. When you are out for a stroll, say, keep your arms down and close to your sides, palms turned forward with thumbs out, and roll your thumbs back as you walk along. Your shoulders move back. No one will guess you are exercising, and you will probably get compliments on your splendid carriage.

Test your ingenuity to find other means of varying the routine. Window shades or venetian blinds, for example, are splendid allies: raise and lower them several times, each time reaching closer to the top of the window. Quite ordinary household tasks can also provide excellent exercise: pushing a vacuum or a sweeper, making beds, putting away things on high shelves—nothing heavy, though—washing and ironing and hanging out clothes; cleaning windows and mirrors; dusting into corners—in short, any task that makes you reach in order to perform it is good for you.

Because there is the key word: *Reach!*

—to confidence in yourself;

—to strength and vitality;

—to renewed physical and emotional health.

So great was the need for guidance in this field of rehabilitation that those first 10,000 copies of the *Manual* were gone within a few months. A second edition was published the next year, a third the year after that.

An article describing my postoperative experience and urging the establishment of some comprehensive program of therapy appeared in the *New York Journal-American*. Another appeared in the magazine *Coronet* in 1954. The mail response was overwhelming: "I need not tell you how very depressed I am and at times cannot even perform the duties of a mother"; "No one can understand more fully what one goes through, but a woman who has had the experience"; "My doctor is a great surgeon but is so busy I never said much about the emotional problems I was fighting every day"; "I am deeply interested in behalf of my daughter, it has been very difficult for her to consent to this surgery and as the time draws near she is becoming very depressed"; "I agree with you there is a desperate need for understanding and encouragement at a time like this"—the letters came, and kept coming, and it was obvious that even with redoubled effort and a 36-hour day no one person could keep up with the rehabilitation that was crying to be done.

Fortunately for the Reach to Recovery Program, and for me personally, one of the corsetieres with whom I talked during my safaris through the city introduced me to Mrs. Walter Rosenau. This truly remarkable woman had had a mastectomy almost ten years before, and she shared my ardor and determination to be of help to others who had undergone the operation. From the moment of our meeting, the specter of trying to carry on single-handed vanished. Fan Rosenau became my valued colleague and has been so ever since.

Shortly after we began working together, an opportunity arose to speak before a graduating class of nurses in Mississippi. I decided to go. After an overnight trip I checked into a hotel, showered and changed, and arrived at the hospital to find an audience of not only student nurses but several older women as well.

A note was handed to me: "I do so need to have a little talk with you. Please don't ask me to see you here at the hospital. May I come to your hotel? Will explain when I see you." The note was signed "Lottie S.," but who in the crowded room that might be there was no way of guessing.

At the conclusion of the lecture I mentioned casually that I should be at the hotel until nine that evening if anyone wished to talk privately. Then I asked for questions from the audience. One of the older women stood up and introduced herself (the name was not "Lottie S.") . She was a registered nurse, she said, and had had both breasts removed five years before. Since then, she had been unable to raise either of her arms above chest level. She wanted to know whether Reach to Recovery exercises could improve that condition.

Her question posed questions: Had she had complete mobility before her surgery? Yes, she had. Had she had complications at the time of either mastectomy which explained such immobility? No, she had not. In the years since, had anything occurred that would explain it? No, nothing had. There was no reasonable explanation for her having such limited movement—except that she had never been given exercises. And she had never devised any on her own initiative.

Skepticism colored the woman's tone and attitude—she was challenging Reach to Recovery with a problem which she felt sure the Program could not solve. Yet beneath that skepticism was an unmistakable current of desperation. Her work as a nurse was deteriorating, her morale as a woman was dropping steadily; what we in that crowded room were hearing was really a cry for help.

So, there and then, we went to work.

Appropriate exercises were demonstrated, and the next hour was a busy one. For five years—sixty long months—this woman had not raised her arms even shoulder high, and she was convinced it was impossible for her to do so (had her shoulder been "frozen" with calcific deposits, as might have been the case, a speedy correction would have been unlikely; luckily, this was not so) . What had not happened in five years did happen, that afternoon, in sixty minutes—she was raising both arms *because for the first time she was truly trying.* With instruction, encouragement, and the aid of the pulley, she was reaching almost to the top of her head before she left that lecture hall.

During my own struggle back to health, each small physical victory had always given me a tremendous lift. Witnessing the victories of others does the same. I left the hospital that afternoon buoyant and exhilarated.

Somewhat to my surprise, the mysterious "Lottie S." was not waiting at the hotel. Her note had sounded so urgent—yet five o'clock came and went, six o'clock came and went, and she did not appear. I had dinner served in my room so as not to risk missing her.

A few minutes before eight, there was a knock on my door.

For some reason, I had imagined "Lottie S." as quite young, possibly one of the student nurses. She turned out to be a woman in her fifties, a clerical worker and the mother of four daughters. She had been a widow for the past eleven years. Her eldest daughter, Barbara, was now nineteen and a member of the class to whom I had spoken that afternoon.

Lottie explained that she had not wanted to approach me at the meeting for fear of embarrassing her daughter in front of her classmates.

"Embarrassing her?" I was puzzled. "In what way?"

"Well, because," Lottie said, "she's ashamed of this." Her left arm, the side of her operation, was twice the girth of the other, and very "brawny," or hard.

As a nurse, her daughter most likely knew that swelling, or lymphedema, in the affected arm is not uncommon following a mastectomy, and that the extent of the lymphedema varies considerably. But as a student, the chances were that Barbara had not seen many postoperative mastectomy patients.

Lottie shook her head. "Why she's ashamed," she said, "is on account of I let it get to be this bad. She says it's my own fault it's like this so long after my operation." For a moment she seemed on the verge of tears. "If you want to know, I'm ashamed of it myself. I go to buy a new outfit, try to be fitted, what do I find? I wear a size sixteen in dresses, suits, coats, everything fits perfect but that left sleeve. I start to wondering, maybe do these clerks think I'm some kind of a freak?"

With that, tears did come, quietly, and as if they had been held back a long time. I turned away to pour a cup of tea from the pot on my dinner tray and waited for Lottie to regain her composure.

She accepted the tea gratefully. Her doctor, she told me, permitted her to use a mechanically operated sleeve for relief. This device, like other similar machines, is often used in providing temporary relief from post-mastectomy lymphedema of the arm. (One of the noted physicians who addressed the first Symposium on Rehabilitation and Cancer in New York City stated: "In control of edema of the arm, active use and proper positioning assist. If there is persistence of the edema, help can be obtained from mechanical aids and massage as well as exercise.")

If your doctor approves of the use of a mechanical aid, you may find that it sometimes brings a distinct softening of the arm's "brawniness," reduction of "pitting," and a reduction or lessening of pain in your arm or chest. The way it works is simple. Your arm is slipped into the sleeve, the switch is flipped, and treatment is under way. There is no discomfort. Treatment can be given in your doctor's office or, with his approval (the unit is portable), in your own home while you are watching TV or reading or just relaxing. The machine is no cure-all, but it does help some women.

It helped Lottie but, in the opinion of her daughter, not enough. The girl blamed her mother for being remiss about exercising—"And y'know," Lottie said morosely, "to tell the honest truth she's right. Only she never did show me *what* exercises to do, and nobody else did, either." Brawniness had so immobilized her arm that she could no longer use that arm to cook or bake or do housework. Prodded by her daughter and by her own growing concern, she had asked her doctor for permission to receive instruction from me in Reach to Recovery exercises. He had consented at once.

That evening I had a reservation on a 9:47 flight back to New York. I did not make the flight. There was another, two hours later. I missed that one, too.

Weariness was forgotten as Lottie and I went to work there in the hotel room. She was hurting, I could see that, but she did not complain. I warned her not to expect any miracles; it was going to take time, and hard work—time that evening and time over the weeks and months ahead—and *perhaps* the exercises would help. As a guide for keeping up with the regimen on her own, Lottie put a copy of the *Reach to Recovery Manual* in her purse. She examined the assortment of bras and breast forms that I had used for demonstration in my lectures earlier (her own prosthesis was quite inadequate) we selected a few that were suitable for her and I wrote down the name of a local corsetiere who could supply the forms and, hopefully, guarantee the all-important proper fitting.

Finally, I showed Lottie how to "center" her figure in dressing and how to maintain evenness of line in her appearance, and she prepared to leave.

It was well after 11 P.M.

At the door we shook hands warmly. Lottie hesitated, and when she spoke there was a catch in her voice. "What I said before, about being a freak, you forget that, okay?" Her eyes were shining. "What I am," said Lottie, "is a woman same as any other. And for the first time in years, I feel like one!"

So—to sum up—here are seven signposts to watch for along your personal road back to health:

1. Recognize the Reach to Recovery Program as a team effort—your doctor, your nurse, a physiotherapist, a well-trained Volunteer, and yourself, working together for your maximum physical and emotional recovery. *Don't let that team down.*
2. Remember, the key word is *Reach!* Whatever forces you to reach will help restore your strength, your mobility and your self-confidence.
3. With your doctor's approval, begin your exercises as soon as possible after your operation, usually while you are still in the hospital.
4. Begin exercising slowly. Do not tire yourself. *But do keep at them.* If they hurt, breathe deeply, pause, relax —then start again.
5. When you are tempted to postpone exercising, *do not yield to the temptation.* Be persistent, day in and day out. Remind yourself of the rewards of that persistence: your own recovery.
6. Cooperate with your doctor. Do not try to outguess him. Follow his instructions.

7. Remember that you are the same person you always were—*and can become even better!* Say this to yourself. Say it aloud. Over and over. Believe it, for it is so.

A long distance call from Mississippi came to my apartment in New York shortly before Christmas.

The caller was Lottie S.

She was, she told me excitedly, using her arm as she had not been able to use it for years. Lymphedema was still present—exercises had worked no magical reduction in that—but the reduction in brawniness seemed almost magical to Lottie. Not only was she now doing her own housework, but she could cook and bake again.

"So I'm celebrating!" Lottie cried happily. "I'm baking up batches of Christmas cookies for all my neighbors—and a box is on its way to you, special delivery, special handling!"

On Christmas Eve the box arrived. The cookies were delicious. And recalling the joyous sound of Lottie's voice added a special joy to the holiday that year, for all of us.

IV

You and Prayer

To live with dignity and enjoy life . . .

For anyone, surely this means first and foremost having peace of mind. For you, as a mastectomy patient, it means having the serenity that comes with the assurance that in thought and appearance you have been restored to a glowing vitality, able to resume your sexual and social role with your husband and to mother your children with verve and energy.

As one of the speakers at the first Symposium on Rehabilitation and Cancer pointed out: "To be effective, rehabilitation must be a driving force . . . to return a patient with a mastectomy to a feminine state of mind."

The cost to a patient of being denied this was made all too clear by a phone call that wakened me at 2 A.M. one winter night.

What the caller was saying made no sense—either it was a bad connection, or the woman was incoherent. Then a single word jolted me wide awake: "Suicide."

Gathering my wits, "Who is this?" I asked. "Who's calling?"

"Never mind that—"

By now I was out of bed, pulling on a robe.

The voice repeated, "I'm going to commit suicide tonight, Mrs. Lasser."

A thought flashed across my mind: *Those who talk about it don't do it.* On the heels of that, another thought: *Sometimes they do, though.*

"Where are you?" Learn that, I was thinking, and send help before she hangs up. Somehow (but how?) send help. "Where are you calling from?"

The receiver buzzed with a jumble of slurred words, most of them unintelligible, but "my priest" came through clearly, and "a mortal sin," and a name that sounded like "Barney," and a reference to "the last ferry." Ferry? Did that locate her as being on Staten Island? A needle in a haystack. How many hundreds of thousand people lived on Staten Island? And wasn't there another ferry running somewhere else? Where? Where? While I kept the woman talking, part of my mind prayed desperately, *God, show me what to say, what to do!*

Once more I begged her to tell me her name, and this time she did so.

I said gently, "Come to see me in the morning, Anna. Will you do that, please? We'll talk this all out together. I understand how you feel but don't do anything about it until we have a chance to talk, first thing in the morning. Promise me that."

"Barney's gone," Anna said. Her voice had a flattened, empty sound.

"Barney? You mean, your husband?"

"He walked out tonight." Her breath caught in a sob. "He said he wouldn't live with a one-tit bitch, then he walked out."

"Anna, a man who would say such a thing must be—"

"I don't want to live," she said, and hung up.

Was this the answer to my prayer for guidance? Her name and nothing more? But wait—there *was* more: Possibly that the call had come from somewhere on Staten Island, and most probably—from the reference to "my priest" and to suicide as "a mortal sin"—that the caller was a Catholic. It was not much, but it was enough to take up the phone and dial the Rectory at St. Patrick's Cathedral. The time was 2:20 A.M.

A monsignor answered. I explained the situation. If he would supply me with the phone numbers of the parishes on Staten Island, I would call them one after another until—hopefully—the woman's priest was located.

Moments later, on the second call, I was talking to Father H., who knew Anna and her husband, Barney, and was aware of the growing friction in their household since Anna's mastectomy some weeks before. "But I cannot believe Anna would take her own life!" Father H. would nevertheless go to Anna at once. "Did she ask you to call me?"

I told him that Anna had refused even to tell me where she lived.

He sounded bewildered. "Then however did you locate—?"

"With help, Father," I said. "God's help." And the thought came that from the moment I had prayed to be shown what to do and had, in effect, put the crisis in His hands, I had known that one way or another He *would* help.

It has happened that way so often.

Again and again I, who am not religious in a churchgoing sense, have found the power of prayer to be truly awesome. It has been called the most enormous energy source in the universe, and that, beyond a doubt, is true. Again and again the unsolvable has become, for me, solved through prayer. "Man ought always to pray," Luke tells us, "and not to faint." Writing to the Romans, Paul declared that "All things work together for good to them that love God"—and how very carefully Paul phrased that, and how truly, because things *do* work for our good when we love God, and He allows each of us to work with Him through love, and share that good.

I believe that no one's destiny is preordained. The life we live in this world is what we make of it, each of us, individually, provided only that we abide by the logic of His laws for orderliness in life. We are creatures of free will with a precious spark of Him within to alert us to the good He has made available to us.

Without that spark and without His guidance, I believe that I could never have brought the Reach to Recovery Program into being.

His design for us is good. Evil has intruded upon that design in many forms—fear, ignorance, hate, anxiety and pain, illness and disease—but we need not be Evil's passive victims. Indeed, we must not be. God, who owes us nothing, yet gives us everything that is good, asks in return only that we collaborate with Him in making the utmost of his most precious gift to us—ourselves. To achieve this, He will provide us with a helping hand, but we are expected to stand upon our own two feet. This, I believe, is the only way to achieve the ultimate in physical and mental well-being.

Ask, and it shall be given you—yes, but not served up without effort on our part.

Seek, and ye shall find—yes, by putting to use the five senses He gave us with which to seek, and to find.

Knock, and it shall be opened unto you—yes, provided we reach out and tug the latchstring with our own hands.

Acceptance of this relationship with God can become the

foundation for that inner serenity and peace of mind which is so essential to living with dignity and enjoying life.

And "When you love," the mystic Kahlil Gibran tells us, "you should not say, 'God is in my heart,' but rather 'I am in the heart of God.' "

Dawn was lightening the sky when Father H. called back. He had arrived at Anna's house to find an emptied bottle of sleeping pills, and Anna in a coma. He had phoned her doctor, who summoned an ambulance. Father H. rode to the hospital with Anna. She had been given emergency treatment, and her condition was listed as critical.

Was there anything at all I could do to help this poor woman?

"Pray for her," the priest said quietly, "and God's will be done."

Pray . . . and God's will be done.

But how difficult it is, sometimes, to comprehend His will and to accept it.

Was it His will, for instance, that while Reach to Recovery was still in its formative stage my husband should suffer a third, and fatal, heart attack? I have come to think that had he survived, my husband would have had to adapt to a sluggish pace of living, which for such a man would have been intolerable, and that God in His wisdom knew that. But at the time I knew only that my beloved companion and most loyal friend had been taken from me, and in my grief I rebelled against accepting that loss or trying to comprehend it.

It was not God who denied me His comfort during that period, but I who denied it to myself.

Instead, I threw myself into my work, recruiting and training Volunteers, writing magazine articles about Reach to Recovery, talking to doctors and nurses and physiotherapists, expanding the annual Open Forum concept for exchange of ideas and dissemination of information, visiting patients in hospitals, lecturing whenever and wherever anyone would listen. And I was interviewed on radio and television by Mike Douglas, Virginia Graham, Arlene Francis, Martha Deane, and many many others.

Knowing that most women who heard these broadcasts had not had a mastectomy, I always made it a point to stress the importance of self-examination of the breast; listeners were urged to write to the American Cancer Society for a leaflet describing the technique of breast self-examination.

In spite of the fact that in the decade between 1960 and 1970 public knowledge about cancer has shown a notable increase, the American Cancer Society in 1971 reported a leveling off in the number of individuals motivated to take specific action, such as annual checkups. The Society emphasized the high lifesaving potential of regular self-examination in the incidence of breast cancer, and stressed to women that 95 percent of patients discover a lump in their breast themselves through such self-examination.

The technique is simple. Do make it a habit, as routine as brushing your hair or giving yourself a facial or a manicure—except that a breast check need be done only once a month, immediately following your menstrual period.

You may find it convenient to begin while you're bathing, when your fingers will slide easily across your wet skin. Keeping your fingers flat, gently touch every area of your breasts, feeling for any lump or thickening. The chances are that you will feel nothing in the least unusual—and if you do, the chances are it is no cause for alarm at all. As you check the lower part of your breasts, do not be surprised if you feel a firm ridge—that, as a rule, is perfectly normal.

Next, sit before a mirror with your arms down at your sides, and look for any dimpling in the skin or changes in the nipples. Then raise your arms and look for the same thing.

Finally, lie down with a pillow beneath your left shoulder, bend your left arm back to place your hand under your head. With the fingers of your right hand flattened to the skin at the outer edge of your left breast, circle your hand slowly and gently inward toward the nipple in a spiralling, clockwise movement. Shift the pillow under your right shoulder, put your right hand back beneath your head, and examine your left breast in the same way. To be absolutely thorough, sit up and repeat the procedure once more.

That's all there is to it—a few moments invested once each month in doing the best thing possible to protect yourself.

It is important to perform this breast self-examination regularly. And should you discover a lump, see your doctor. And don't panic—most lumps or changes in the breast are simply cysts or harmless tumors; of those that are biopsied, about eight out of ten are benign.

One day I arrived home to find a florist's box reposing on the drop-leaf table. In it were a dozen exquisite roses and a note: "Because our prayers have been answered." The note was signed "Mr. and Mrs. C.K.N."

The name was unfamiliar: Mr. and Mrs. C.K.N.? Who were they? What prayers of theirs had been answered? And whyever send me roses because of it?

The next day Mr. and Mrs. C.K.N. called in person.

They were in their sixties, soft-spoken, shy, with that kind of quietly happy rapport between them to which strangers warm instinctively. When Mr. N. said something, he would glance quickly at his wife for confirmation. When Mrs. N. said something, she would look to her husband in the same way. The impression they gave was of two people who, through years of a good marriage, had in fact become one and were highly satisfied that that was the case.

They explained the prayers that had been answered, and the reason for the roses.

Their elder daughter, Kitty, just forty, had been living with them since her husband's death eight years before. The past winter, she had made plans to remarry. Then she discovered a lump in her breast. Their family doctor sent her to a surgeon, who recommended a biopsy. Kitty flatly refused. Not only would she not consent to a biopsy; she was by then refusing to concede that there was a lump at all.

"No amount of talking would budge her," Mr. N. said, glancing at his wife.

"The doctor said that a biopsy was absolutely a must," Mrs. N. said, nodding. "I begged her to have it. Her father begged her. Her sister begged her." She looked at her husband, who nodded.

"George tried to get her to listen to reason," Mr. N. said. "George, that's her fiancé, a fine man, told Kitty it wouldn't change a thing even if it turned out she had to have a—a—"

"Mastectomy," Mrs. N. said. "But Kitty wouldn't budge."

The family doctor had spelled it out for Kitty: Her life was at stake. Kitty's response was that if she had to die, she would die with two breasts, not one.

"What do you do with a girl like that?" Mr. N. said. "Old enough to know better, have some sense, but no. Got so's she wouldn't even discuss it at all, just up and left the room if anybody so much as looked as if the subject was coming up."

"We've never been what you'd call a religious family," Mrs. N. said softly, glancing at her husband. He shook his head.

"We don't go to church," he said, "and we're not much for prayers. Anyhow, I never was."

"But when absolutely nothing would budge Kitty," Mrs. N. said, "what else was left but prayer?"

"I'll be honest," Mr. N. said, "Before this, if I ever thought about God at all, it was to doubt that there was any such being, or power, or whatever name you want to give Him."

Doubts notwithstanding, they had prayed together for their daughter.

"It wasn't so much praying, like in church," Mrs. N. said. "We just sat at the table and folded our hands and closed our eyes, and we just sort of talked to Him, as if He was in the room with us, and said please, would He help Kitty."

Mr. N. said, "Frankly, I didn't see what God could do about it. I mean, to change Kitty's mind. I mean, how could He? Speak to her in a dream? Send down an angel? Frankly, I just didn't see it."

"All the same," Mrs. N. said, "we did it." Her husband nodded, and for a moment they were both silent, remembering. Then, "The very next morning," Mrs. N. said in a hushed tone, "we were working in the kitchen, Kitty and I. It was a few minutes after ten. Kitty never listens to the radio, but that morning she switched it on."

"To the Martha Deane show," Mr. N. said, nodding.

Mrs. N. said, "Somebody was talking, and it was you, Mrs. Lasser. Kitty stopped what she was doing, and listened. You were saying that if these things are caught early and diagnosed and treated, that's half the battle. And you sounded so confident, so brimful of life. I watched Kitty. She went pale, then her color began to come back. She didn't look at me. It was as if I wasn't there in the room at all, just you two alone, and she paid attention like she never had to any of us."

"She not only paid attention," Mr. N. said, "she changed her mind. Decided her doctor and the surgeon were right, and checked into the hospital that same night. The biopsy showed cancer, so she had a mastectomy."

"She's home now," Mrs. N. said happily. "The doctors say it was caught early enough, they couldn't be more optimistic, so you see our prayers were answered in more ways than one."

"And the wedding," Mr. N. said, "is still set for June."

When they left, I thought about what Mr. N. had said—that prior to this experience, if he ever thought about God at all, it was to doubt His existence.

Do you, at this moment in your life? Do you, too, doubt?

Now, when you so desperately need the reassurance of His love, can you expect to find a truly personal God, responsive to that need, responsive to you as an individual?

Or is such an expectation unrealistic? Is His existence, in fact, merely a myth?—a holdover from a long past time to which none of us can ever return?

"We can never actually define God," says Joshua Loth Liebman in his best seller, *Peace of Mind,* "since we human beings are so limited and our language is always inexact, and we shall probably always have to use metaphor and analogy in order to interpret divine reality." On the vaulted ceiling of the Sistine Chapel, in Rome, Michelangelo chose to interpret divine reality as an all-powerful, graybearded father figure. In the Old Testament He is interpreted as being "Merciful and gracious, long-suffering, and abundant in goodness and truth." (Exodus 34) In the New Testament,

He is "Love, and he that dwelleth in love dwelleth in God, and God in him." (I John 4) A noted theologian, Mordecai Kaplan, defines Him, in part, thus:

God is in the faith
By which we overcome
The fear of loneliness, of helplessness,
Of failure and of death.

God is in the hope
Which, like a shaft of light,
Cleaves the dark abysms
Of sin, of suffering, of despair.

God is in the love
Which creates, protects, forgives.

It seems to me that it is perhaps enough to say simply that *If we have God, He exists.*

Surely there is no irreverence in interpreting divine reality as a close and constant companion. "We just sort of talked to Him, as if He was in the room with us," Mrs. N. had said. And the very next morning her daughter, who never listened to the radio, had switched it on and listened, and her mind, which had been made up, was changed. . . .

During your own time of crisis, when it is so easy to feel forsaken and lost, try talking to Him as if He were in the room with you. Try putting your feelings into words and saying the words aloud. Speak to Him simply and forthrightly, as you would to a trusted and intimate friend.

I have talked to Him in just that way—and found Him to be both personal and responsive.

In the early days of Reach to Recovery it was a struggle to

find the funds to keep the Program alive. Working out of the apartment eliminated the overhead of an office, and the generosity to Mrs. Rosenau and to me of family and friends, and grateful patients, helped defray other expenses. But as the Program grew and expanded, so did its costs. If help had not come to us from somewhere, we could not have continued.

And help did come—always timely, always in the way it was most urgently needed. Was it simply coincidence, when costs mounted on the Dacron fluff for the breast forms so vital to our kits, that through a volunteer, Rose O'Connor, the Dupont Company began delivering it free of charge? Or that the manufacturer of these breast forms, Walter J. Kautsch Enterprises, in Detroit, steadfastly refused to bill us for them? Or that costly equipment such as typewriters was made less costly for us by IBM? Or that John Van Derwerken of Baronet Litho, in Johnstown, New York, for sixteen years did all our printing, on the finest of papers, and never accepted payment for a line of it?

Was it all coincidence? Or was it prayers being answered? *All things work together for good to them that love God*—again and again that wonderful truth has been affirmed for us at the Reach to Recovery Program. Progress in the field of rehabilitation for the cancer patient is such affirmation. So are the advances in early detection such as mammography and thermography.

With physical examination still the mainstay of detecting breast cancer, and most lumps still discovered by the patients themselves through self-examination, the American Cancer Society also encourages the use of mammography (X-ray examination of the breasts) when facilities are available and when advised by the examining physician. This technique can be impressively accurate in detecting cancers that may be too small to be discovered by palpation; such early detection dramatically increases the possibility of cure.

Thermography, a heat-pattern technique of detection of cancer, is also useful and likewise requires specially trained operating personnel. In general the medical centers in the larger cities have the necessary equipment. Hopefully, mammography and thermography will become more available so that they can be used in conjunction with the physician's examination to move yet closer to that all-important goal of early, *early* detection of breast cancer.

V

You and Your Family

THE SUAVE MANAGER checks his appointments list.

"Ah! Yes! Mrs. Crowther. Two-thirty. Facial, rinse, and set, *oui,* madame?"

The customer nods, glancing toward the curtained booths in the rear.

The manager looks less suave and makes odd clucking sounds. "Mrs. Crowther, *je me suis trompé*—a mistake has been made, you asked for Paul, *je suis navré,* there will be a delay—" His face brightens. "Ah! But Albert! Albert will be free momentarily, madame."

The customer shrugs. "Anyone will do." She smiles. "He'd better know his business, that's all—heavens, it's been fourteen years since I set foot inside a beauty shop!" She adds, without saying it aloud, "And I wouldn't be here now, except for my operation."

The Paul-Albert beauty shop is fictitious. So is the customer. But there is nothing fictitious about the thousands of women like Mrs. Crowther who, after their operations, set about creating exciting new images of themselves—spurred to do so, more often than not, by the Reach to Recovery Program of the American Cancer Society, whose aim is to improve the life of the patient who has had a mastectomy.

It is a phenomenon that we at Reach to Recovery witness often: A mastectomy patient, fearful of becoming less feminine, tends to become *more* feminine, more meticulous about her person, dressing with care and grooming herself (with or without an assist from a beauty shop) so that her entire image as a woman becomes enormously attractive and in many respects more stunning than ever before.

It is as though her brush with a serious illness has opened the woman's eyes to a new appreciation of life, and of herself.

When the time comes for *you* to leave the hospital to return home, do let this new appreciation of life show itself to those around you. Make a conscious effort to project an attractive image of yourself. Fix your hair so it looks its best. Touch color to your cheeks. Wear a smile, and think thoughts that will make the smile genuine. So that the site of the operation will look as normal as possible, wear your breast form from the Reach to Recovery Kit in a lounge bra or your own bra with an extender.

Carry away with you from the hospital the conviction that your postoperative recovery is going to be the beginning of a new and more positive life.

That phrase—*the beginning of a new and more positive life*—I first heard some years ago from a patient in Cleveland, Ohio. The youngest of a large family, Alice Q. was unmarried and living at home with parents who treated her more like a carefree child than a mature, thirty-two-year-old woman.

Her father, for instance, budgeted her wages. Her mother selected her wardrobe. Her four brothers and two sisters, all married, thought of her still as "the baby of the family," and Alice wrote that she had never in her entire life made a really important decision or handled a really serious responsibility. "To be honest, I sort of enjoyed being spoiled and catered to. Anyhow, if anybody'd asked me, I'd have said I enjoyed it."

Needless to say, when Alice underwent a mastectomy, there was no lack of familial attention.

But for once that attention had little meaning. Alice was learning what it was to be alone.

Then, "While in the hospital," she wrote, "I met a woman who received such a shock—she was coming out of the anaesthesia when she overheard her doctor telling her husband that her breast had been removed. Before I knew the details I thought she looked most unhappy and wondered what caused such a look about her eyes." When they became acquainted, the woman confided to Alice the nightmare of her awakening and the terror that still gripped her, and her fears about the future. "Then at least once a day she would come to my room, we would compare notes and I tried to cheer her up by being positive, so to speak. When she came to say goodbye, she looked a great deal happier (if I may use the word) and no doubt it had helped her to speak to another in the same condition."

Instead of being dependent, Alice had found herself being depended upon. And rising to that responsibility, she found the experience exhilarating. A side of Alice Q.'s character no one suspected began to emerge.

Her letter continued, "My sister Rose (she meant well) made a great mistake by writing a short note on a get-well card—it was just oozing sympathy, and that did not set too well with me. Then Mother came to see me, with my other sister, Edie. They brought gifts, and when I took a little too long to open the bows, Mother and Edie wanted to help me—that was another mistake! I did not and do not want to be made to feel helpless."

Very much a new Alice, with a new attitude toward herself and a new appreciation of life. Her letter concluded, "If I should meet some wonderful man, there will be the problem of telling him, but I am sure that will work out all right. I am sure this is the beginning of a new and more positive life for me."

Repeat those words to yourself: *This is the beginning of a new and more positive life.* Say them again and again. They will provide an anchor for your morale at a time when you can use an anchor—the return home after a mastectomy is a serious emotional challenge. It is a strain, facing your family's anxiety and love when you are so vulnerable, when your confidence can so easily be undermined by too much sympathy or solicitude—or, worst of all, expressions of pity.

This is not the time for heroics on your part. Certainly you have earned the right to the healing catharsis of tears, and if emotion is overwhelming and it helps to give way and weep for yourself a little, by all means do so. Only remember that you have faced a far greater challenge than this one, and triumphed over it—*you are alive.*

Remember, too, that for a while you will be very much center stage at home. What you do, what you say, how you act will be your family's cues for what to do and say, and how to act. Make the most of this concern by giving as good as you receive: Accept solicitude, but do not make a crutch of it; accept help, but never exploit it; and try always to bear in mind that the best room freshener of all is cheerfulness.

It should not surprise you if no one at home is quite at ease with you at first. There are few perils so jolting to a family as the threatened loss of a beloved member, and for some crucial hours recently your family did face that peril. It is behind them now, happily, but it will have left its mark. Your husband and your children can be expected to have a highly charged awareness of you as wife and mother for some while to come.

Especially do not underestimate what this time of peril has meant to your husband.

My leaflet, "A Letter to Husbands," which is included in Reach to Recovery Kits, says about homecomings, "There is a difficult period of adjustment." That might be expanded to read "mutually difficult" because just as aching doubts have tormented you, this man who shares your life has been having some aching doubts, himself.

Nothing erases such doubts faster than a desire on his part to put them to rest.

His sympathy, his understanding, his positive attitude toward the future are what will do the most to speed his wife—you—to full emotional and physical recovery and so hasten a return to normal for the family and the man himself.

"Barriers are created," "A Letter to Husbands" goes on, "by changes in previously existing patterns when these changes are interpreted as the result of the physical disability." As has already been stressed, if a part of the existing pattern of your marriage has been your husband seeing you dress and undress, a barrier will be created if he now alters that pattern by leaving the room at such times. He may be showing sympathy by doing so, but his wife, you, may interpret this as showing distinct distaste for the sight of her. Any woman needs to be assured of two things at her homecoming: 1) that she has been missed, and 2) that she is still wanted. A noted psychiatrist speaking before an American Cancer

Society-sponsored conference on rehabilitation put it this way: "A husband who is encouraged to grin lecherously at his wife on her return home from the hospital will do more than any occupational therapy program can do." (And do bear in mind that your role as a woman calls upon you to do your feminine part to stimulate that lecherous grin!)

Not long ago I was waiting to board my flight after a lecture before a group in Lansing, Michigan. The airport was fogged in, there had already been two postponements of takeoff, and cancellation of the flight seemed imminent. Phone booths were jammed with agitated passengers making hasty changes in plans.

A man at one of the phones completed his call, burst out of the booth and collided with me.

"Sorry! Clumsy of me! Are you all right?"

The collision, I assured him, had been minor.

He was looking at me intently. "Say! Aren't we old friends? Of course we are!"

We had never met, as far as I could recall.

But he was pumping away at my hand as though we were in fact long lost friends. "The world shrinks, eh? Two years ago. We worked together. Tel-Aviv!"

Then I remembered. . . .

On that visit to Tel-Aviv, the Israel Cancer Association had suggested that part of the usual Reach to Recovery demonstration be bypassed. So many Israeli women have Oriental backgrounds, I was told, that they would never come forward in an open meeting to be fitted with one of our temporary prostheses. In fact, it was strongly hinted that no women would attend the meeting at all.

But they did, many accompanied by their husbands. And they remained for hours, being shown exercises, being fitted, while the men not only asked penetrating questions but learned the exercises and helped their wives to do them.

One of the husbands who had worked most patiently with his wife was this man in the fogbound Michigan airport.

"How is she now?" I was beginning to recall her as a woman who had been operated on years prior to that meeting and who had never regained full use of her arm on the side of the operation.

"A new woman!" Her husband laughed. "That experience began a change for the better in our lives, in more ways than one."

His love and tenderness, I assured him, his patience and eagerness to help, above all his *being there,* had played a very important part in making of his wife "a new woman."

And suddenly, as if a camera clicked in my mind, I saw her clearly: a wisp of a woman, quite pretty, wide-eyed and soft-spoken, who must have had discomfort and even pain in doing the exercises, but had not flinched from them at all. And they had given her, there on the spot, more mobility than she had had in years.

An hour later, with her husband, she had been waiting in the lobby.

When I came down the stairs she stepped forward, holding out a tiny bunch of fresh violets.

She spoke no English. I spoke no Hebrew. But as she gently pressed the little flowers into my hand there were tears in her eyes, and no words were necessary for either of us.

Volunteers of the Reach to Recovery Program find that many patients wish to include their husbands in the sessions—and that husbands wish to be included. As a matter of fact, men frequently ask more far-reaching questions, more frankly, than do their wives. And for a woman to witness on the part of her husband this genuine concern for her physical and mental well-being is the soundest kind of therapy.

More than anyone else, it is your husband who can make you feel needed and wanted. And by doing this he will not only help you regain confidence as a woman and as a wife, but he will be displaying the stature of his manhood.

So—again summing up—for the husband whose wife has recently returned home after this operation, or will soon be coming home, here are six suggestions to help you through this difficult period of adjustment:

1. Be understanding—but do not be overly solicitous, because that could encourage morbid self-pity. Try to banish the words *ashamed* and *inferior* from her vocabulary. Make her know she is a woman, not an invalid.

2. Love her. Say the word to her. L O V E. Say it often. Show it by affectionate interest in her as an individual. The richness of her femininity is still there, all of it, waiting to respond.

3. Reassure her. Tell her that she has a hidden scar and nothing more—that no one need know of it unless she chooses to tell. She is the same person she's always been. Tell her that, too. Often.

4. Be kind. If it has been your custom to be present when she is dressing, do not shut a door between you. Do not leave the room when she is undressing. Be tender. Be natural. Above all, *be there.*

5. Resume the sexual relationship. Nothing that has happened has diminished her ability to love. The better the relationship within a marriage, the less its depen-

dence upon the partners' physical endowments. Resume the relationship. Soon.

6. Be sympathetic—give her encouragement, patience and compassion in equal parts. Add a dollop or two of good humor because one shared smile can be a more eloquent message of understanding and love than a hundred words.

"What got to me more than anything else," said Mrs. C.B., "was the look in their eyes. Like they thought my days were numbered for sure."

A group of us were relaxing at the Reach to Recovery office after one of the regular monthly sessions of Volunteers for practice and discussion; the talk had turned to our families' reactions when we had returned home following our operations.

"I fooled them," Mrs. C.B. went on. "It's been three years and I feel better than ever."

Although the American Cancer Society emphasizes that Reach to Recovery is not a club and never has been, there is often a warm rapport and a sense of fellowship among its Volunteers, whose dedication is, of course, the very backbone of the rehabilitation work.

Miss O'L. said, "I honestly never think of my operation at all, only when I bathe or shower. But my parents have never stopped thinking about it, I guess. *I'm* the one who has to keep cheering *them* up."

One of the prime requisites for becoming a Volunteer is emotional stability. These women not only had that, but also positive points of view.

"An adjustment I didn't have to make," Mrs. M.K. said,

"was with a husband. I've been separated from my children's father for twelve years."

Someone asked how many children Mrs. M.K. had.

"Three. All boys. Twenty-two, twenty, and going on nineteen. And they've been just wonderful through this whole thing."

"In what way, 'wonderful'?" I wanted to know. Attitudes of children of both sexes are so important to a mother at this time. And not only to her—they affect the climate of the entire household.

Mrs. M.K. thought a moment. "Well," she said, "they took it in stride, that's all." Her sons had been tender, she added, but not too tender. And helpful, but never too helpful. "They just would not let me feel sorry for myself, not for one minute." She laughed suddenly. "We really have a lot of fun over the falsies. I have the inflated form, and the boys take turns offering to blow it up with their football pump!"

They took it in stride.

Instinctively those three young men had adopted exactly the right attitude to help their mother make this most difficult of adjustments.

No teen-age son, however, should expect such an adjustment to occur overnight. He should realize that it will not be easy, and that Mother's grit and courage in achieving it will be helped immeasurably by his own understanding approach to the situation.

But what, exactly, is an understanding approach? A new Reach to Recovery leaflet, "A Letter to a Son," explores this idea.

For one thing, it is taking Mother less for granted. It is being more than usually tuned in to her likes and dislikes, her needs, her emotional ups and downs. No son should go overboard about this—a very *wrong* approach would be to encourage Mother to feel sorry for herself. Simply be natural. Be matter-of-fact. But add a little extra measure of consideration, a little extra show of affection. Masculine strength is at its best when it is being most gentle and patient with someone of the opposite sex, and for quite a while to come Mother will appreciate the gift of gentleness and patience from you, her son.

A letter came to Reach to Recovery from a woman who wrote, "I grew up in a highly emotional family—all of us wore our hearts on our sleeves, so to speak. When my surgeon said that sometimes relatives hinder a patient's recovery with sympathy, pity or even out-and-out grief, I knew my parents and sisters and brothers would do exactly that. So my daughter is the only one who knows I had the operation. She is only fifteen, but mature for her age and she has been so thoughtful and helpful to me."

So thoughtful and helpful.

In uniquely personal ways, a teen-age daughter can be most helpful to Mother at this time. She should know, for example, that there is nothing Mother needs more right now than constant reminders of her own femininity. Provide those reminders, as only you, her daughter, can. How? By talking clothes with her, from her point of view; by helping her to be with it about styles in fashions and cosmetics, from her point of view; by sparing the time from your own preoccupations to go shopping together.

Assume that Mother is the same person she has always been, because, in truth, she is. Nothing has changed except that she now must wear a breast form. Unless she chooses to tell, no one will know about it—and with a bit of fixing up here and adding to there, she will be able to wear almost everything in her wardrobe—including swimsuits.

Be sparing with the sympathy (encouraging Mother toward self-pity is doing her no favor) but be generous with those many small attentions which say to her so clearly, "I love you, Mom."

It was once believed that cancer in a family could be inherited, particularly breast cancer. The fact is, it is not inherited in the true sense; there is, though, evidence of an increased possibility of its occurrence in a family with a strong history of breast cancer. This should not be alarming. It simply means that early detection of a change or a lump in the breast becomes doubly important. This extra precaution more often than not benefits a girl's over-all health. A spokesman for the American Cancer Society states that "Although breast cancer is usually found in women of middle age and over . . . the Society recommends that efforts also be directed toward educating girls of high school age"—because early detection is so vital that monthly breast self-examination (page 66) should become a habit in the teens.

Our Reach to Recovery leaflet "To Someone Special" reminds a daughter to "remember that the normal and easy acceptance of your mother, as a person, is one of the fastest ways of helping her. By being matter-of-fact, honest and understanding, you will fulfill your mother's real need. Give her your young and loving strength. Your mother will rejoice in it. Both of you will be able to forget the operation in a reasonably short time and to be closer than before."

The leaflet concludes that "This is the time for simple warmth and understanding . . . never pity . . . only love."

To sum up, then, for a teen-ager whose mother has undergone a mastectomy—you are important to her maximum recovery and here is a six-point formula for doing your part to help her to attain that goal:

1. Be more than usually considerate of her comfort, more than usually aware of her likes and dislikes.
2. Be matter-of-fact and natural. Do not fuss over her. Just pay a bit of added attention to her needs.
3. Show her affection. Show her you love her. Help her when she needs your help—but do not make her feel helpless.
4. If you are a boy, be attentive and gently protective in the small, everyday ways that are the evidence of true male strength.
5. If you are a girl, find ways to make her aware of her womanhood. Talk with her about clothes, hers and your own. And about your dating. And about your feminine hopes and dreams.
6. And, boy or girl, include her in your problems and the triumphs of your young life. She is Mother still, and the sooner she resumes the privileges and the responsibilities of that important role in the family, the better for her—and yourself.

VI

You and the Art of Grooming

Three-tenths of a woman's good looks are due to nature, seven-tenths to dress.

—ANCIENT CHINESE PROVERB

THE OFFICE reflected its occupant—large, imposing, cool, efficient. Across a gleaming expanse of desk top I was facing this doctor, some years ago, with no idea of why he had asked me to come to see him while I was in Detroit.

A truly great surgeon, Dr. W. had never welcomed the Reach to Recovery Program with open arms. Knowing how demands on the medical profession were increasing, we had emphasized the pluses of the Program's service to so busy a man—recommending it to his patients would save him and his staff precious time, without cost and without interfering with the doctor-patient relationship.

But no one from Reach to Recovery had yet been summoned to see a patient of Dr. W.'s.

Was I there in his office that day, at his invitation, because he had finally decided to put the Program's service to the test? It seemed unlikely. His conversation thus far had been in generalities—about the public's attitude toward cancer being too defeatist, about the fatality rate being too often publicized when what should be stressed was the rising survival rate; but nothing whatsoever about Reach to Recovery.

Suddenly he leaned forward. "You'll be in town until when, may I ask?"

I explained that the purpose of my visit was to train Volunteers, which usually meant a stay of three or four days.

"While you're here, could you find time to see my wife?"

Coming from Dr. W., it was a curious request. Why did he wish me to see his wife?

"Six years ago," Dr. W. said, "Nelle had a mastectomy." He hesitated, frowning. "She tells me that since her operation she has never really felt that she looked—well, natural, so to speak."

He opened a drawer and placed before him on the desk a copy of the *Reach to Recovery Manual.* On that wide expanse of uncluttered mahogany it seemed postage-stamp small and insignificant. But Dr. W. was eying it thoughtfully.

"A friend showed this to my wife." His gaze came up to meet mine. "Frankly, Mrs. Lasser, I have never counted myself among your most avid admirers."

Yes, I was aware of that.

"Nobody has to sell me on postoperative rehabilitation," Dr. W. said firmly. "But just as my responsibility is the central problems of this disease and its biological management, I say, Leave rehabilitation problems to the professionals." He riffled the pages of the *Manual.* "Nevertheless, Nelle insists that this has been immensely helpful to her. After six years I should not suppose she needed help. But if she says she does, she does."

I wrote down the address of my hotel. "If you'll ask Mrs. W. to call me, Doctor, any morning before eight or after six in the evening, we'll set a time to get together."

One can only guess at the number of women who, as Nelle

W. stated the problem to me later, have never quite achieved a "natural look" after their operations. Their letters about this are poignant and moving: "I have gone to a number of corsetieres and still feel unhappy about the bra given me"; "I'm self-conscious about the fit of my bra. Have a surgical pad, and still one is larger than the other"; "Have been fitted but one goes up and the other down"; "The problem I have as yet been unable to solve is the bra creeping up"; "There is that terrible off-balance feeling, and 'it' is up to my chin. What can be done or where can one go?"—each an echo of heartache, as well as a reminder that without a correctly fitted prosthesis self-confidence is undermined and a "natural look" simply cannot be achieved.

A prosthesis should do three things for a woman: first, give weight to the side of the operation, thus holding down the bra; second, go around a little on the side, and on the top when necessary, thus helping to take the place of the lost muscles; third, give her back her figure. Unless it does all three, it is not fulfilling its purpose.

Long before I saw her, Nelle W. should have had such a prosthesis. A worry of six years' duration was erased in the few hours it took us at Reach to Recovery to show her how to get herself properly fitted and thus achieve a "natural look."

But to expect your first, temporary prosthesis to provide this naturalness is unrealistic. Just try to make of this an effective camouflage until healing is complete.

Wait for your doctor's approval before undertaking to wear your regular bra. Sew a 3-inch piece of elastic into one of your bras onto the back end of the shoulder strap on your affected side; this will provide more "give," and add to your comfort. If wearing a lightweight breast form, sew a V-shaped piece of elastic (with at least three inches space at the widest part of the V) on the bottom of the bra in front, long enough to be hooked onto your girdle at the point of the V. Sometimes it is more comfortable to have a second V on the side or back of the bra.

Just make sure this elastic is long enough—otherwise you will have a feeling of the bra tugging down, which is detrimental to posture as well as to comfort. Another thing you can do is buy a bra extender in a five-and-dime store. This will add another few inches to the width of the bra for extra comfort at this time.

When the time comes for you to be fitted for a permanent weighted breast form (a time, of course, determined only by your doctor), your own comfort demands the very best that you can afford—which doesn't necessarily mean the most expensive form available. The better the fit of your prosthesis, the better your chances of wearing most of your present wardrobe without major alterations.

(Incidentally, look into your medical insurance: a few policies may pay for surgical prostheses, and such items as breast forms and bras with pockets may be tax-deductible when their total cost and other medical expenses exceed a certain percent of your income. When purchasing such items, be sure that the bills are marked "surgical.")

You have a choice of materials from which to select your breast form: real rubber, spun rubber, liquid, silicone, or air. Most are so effective that your choice becomes simply a matter of personal preference. Some department stores stock prosthetic devices, and many shops specialize in them. Your Reach to Recovery Kit contains a list of such sources, some in your area and others from which you may order by mail. Or contact your local unit of the American Cancer Society for assistance—or go to a good corsetiere who has had experience in this line. If you wish, your Reach to Recovery Volunteer will show you how to fashion a weighted or unweighted form of your own.

What is of prime importance is how well you are fitted—so make your selection with great care. Be sure to get as close a match to your natural breast as possible—*on the sides* as well as the *front* and *top*.

A proper fit depends, mostly, upon the expertise of your fitter. There are some details, however, you will have to manage on your own:

1. Be wary of a fitter who takes your bra in one hand, the pocket of your breast form in the other, and goes off somewhere to sew them together. These must be marked or pinned on the spot, before stitching together, to help assure a good fit. Even a fraction of an inch off in any direction (up, down, either side) will be ruinous to comfort and make you aware of wearing a prosthesis, which you should not be.

2. Your bra will fit better, as a rule, if each shoulder strap is brought as close as possible to the shoulder blades. In addition to improving the fit, this will give you an increased feeling of security.

3. If you are accustomed to wearing a long-line bra with wide shoulder straps, lengthen the straps on the needed side, cutting them at the shoulder seams and inserting ½ inch or 1 inch of elastic the same width as the strap. This helps prevent your form from riding up. (Experiment with this on your own, to find the maximum in comfort and efficiency for yourself.)

To achieve a "natural look" in dressing your figure, it is essential to begin by centering. This means that the *space from the front center of your body to each breast must be identical in width, and on an even line.* Do, always, check for this in your mirror. Do not look down at yourself. Look into the mirror to judge your fit. If an uneven line results, say, because you cannot bear the heaviness of a weighted breast form (or are simply more comfortable with a lighter weight) you can usually restore the necessary evenness of line by anchoring your bra down with a piece of V-shaped elastic, the open ends of the V to be at least 2 inches apart at the top. Hook the bottom, closed end of the V to your girdle on the needed side. Perhaps a second piece of V-shaped elastic may be needed in the back or side on the same side.

Being fitted for a permanent prosthesis, incidentally, does not call for replenishing your bureau drawer with an all-new supply of bras. You can utilize many of your old bras by sewing a pocket the approximate size of the breast form on the inside of each bra. The pocket should have snaps on one side, plus a small pleat to accommodate the front depth of the form.

If you are sensitive under your affected arm, and pocket snaps there present a problem to your comfort, consider moving the snaps from the pocket's upper part to the lower, away from the area which is sensitive.

For that matter, pockets can be made without any snaps at all. Patterns for these, in whatever size bra you are wearing, may be secured through the Reach to Recovery Program of your local unit of the American Cancer Society, as may the patterns for the crescent-shaped pads that are so helpful, esthetically, in filling out the hollow above your breast area and around your arm. These come in various sizes. When you wear a tailored suit, sewing one under the lining will improve the fit. You can snap the pad under the strap of the bra, as some women do; others insert it in a pocket in their slips. Many tell us they find this pad helpful with their soft dresses as well as with suits, and you may decide you agree. There is a new bra which will save you the sewing effort. This bra has pockets which extend up to the shoulder. They can be filled in for the woman who needs this replacement to provide the same unbroken line as on the other side. Information about it is available through your local Reach to Recovery Program of the American Cancer Society.

Someone once said that everything is dangerous to those who are afraid of it.

We who have had this operation know what it is to be afraid. But when surgery has been successful and the prognosis is good, and *then* fear takes over, it means the patient has either been misinformed or has in some way misunderstood the facts of her own situation.

Such a patient was little Miss O'D.

Since the earliest days of the Reach to Recovery Program, Volunteers visit a patient only with her doctor's approval. In those days it was always my custom, when arriving at a hospital, to check with the head nurse for any possible last-minute requests of this nature. Miss O'D.'s name was not on my list of patients to visit that day, nor had her doctor made any last-minute request for me to do so. Both the head nurse and the floor nurse, however, felt that it might help this woman if she and I could be alone together for a while. The head nurse busied herself trying to reach the doctor, who was in the building at the time, to seek his permission to arrange such a meeting.

Miss O'D. was in her forties, with no family and no visitors who had called to see her. All her friends, she had explained to the nurses, were "superstitious kooks" about hospitals—"They walk in, they're scared they'll wind up being carried out feet first!" The floor nurse referred to her fondly as "a real character," an elfin type with a cheery "Irish gift of gab" which had made her a favorite with the staff as well as with the other patients.

But suddenly, and for no apparent reason, Miss O'D. had changed.

Her sunny trust in the doctors and nurses vanished behind a cloud of suspicion. She flatly refused to speak to her surgeon. The "gift of gab" with the nurses and other patients disappeared. She plunged into such a profound depression and became so unresponsive that instead of being ready to be sent home—which her physical condition warranted—she was scheduled for a psychiatric consultation.

Waiting while the nurse was speaking with Miss O'D.'s doctor on the phone, I noticed a woman, long hair in disarray, robe flapping out behind her, coming at a fast clip along the corridor. The impression she gave was of being in blind, headlong flight. The nurse indicated that this was, in fact, Miss O'D., then put down the phone, nodding that her doctor had given permission for me to talk with her.

Quickly, without breaking the woman's stride, I fell into step alongside and slipped my arm through hers. For a moment she continued on, seemingly oblivious of my presence. Then she halted abruptly, stared down at my hand on her arm, and jerked away from it.

"You know," I said quietly, "I've had the same operation."

She looked at me for the first time.

I went on, "Can't we talk for a few minutes?" We were

directly opposite the small examining room where I had placed my equipment. *Coax her in there, into privacy, away from the corridor's activity* . . . "Please," I said gently, "trust me. I want to help. Perhaps I can."

She tensed, wild-eyed, still poised for flight, and a faint sound came from her throat that was half gasp, half sob. I nodded as if I understood, and smiled reassurance. Her eyes squeezed shut, and when she opened them some of the wildness was gone. Within seconds, we were inside the little examining room together.

Wherever her thoughts were (and they obviously were not with me) I proceeded calmly as though I had her full attention: Here was the Reach to Recovery Kit. . . . Here was the exercise rope and the rubber ball on its elastic string . . . this was how to use them. . . . Here was our temporary Dacron fluff form—

In midsentence I broke off.

Soundlessly, her body taut and trembling, Miss O'D. was weeping. Tears can be healing, and perhaps it was time for her to be shedding a few for herself. But as words came tumbling through the tears, this was no simple release of grief and self-pity; it was a bursting dam of pent-up terror verging on hysteria.

But why terror now?

Surgery's dangers were behind her. There had been no postoperative complications. Until a few days ago her spirits had been up, her attitude cheerfully optimistic. Yet now she was afraid, desperately so.

Why?

The answer was slow in coming, but finally it did come.

Ignorance—as it so often is—had been fertile soil for fear. Preparing Miss O'D. to be discharged, her doctor had said that as an outpatient she would be having radiation therapy. Miss O'D. had been stunned. She had no recollection of radiation therapy having been mentioned before. The bright bubble of her self-confidence collapsed. She felt trapped by the unknown: *Radiation!*—for reasons which she herself did not comprehend, the word had terrifying connotations for little Miss O'D.

Of course she should have asked her doctor for an explanation of this therapy, why it was being recommended and of what it consisted. Miss O'D. had not done so. Instead, convinced that some ominous change in her condition was being kept from her, she had retreated behind a wall of distrust and silence where her imagination, uncontrolled by facts, ran riot in picturing the worst.

Understanding too little about her own situation, she had misunderstood too much.

"We have learned how crucial timing and communications are in crisis intervention," declared a noted psychiatrist speaking at an American Cancer Society Symposium on Rehabilitation and Cancer. "Crisis intervention is an active process, not a passive one. If a patient is unable to voice the questions . . . we [must] voice them. . . . This is where rehabilitation begins."

No Reach to Recovery Volunteer ever gives medical advice —on the contrary, the Volunteer is trained as carefully in what *not to say* as in what to say. In talking to Miss O'D. that day, I steered carefully away from talk about treatment, simply assuring her that a radiologist—a doctor—was part of that team effort of her doctor, nurse, physiotherapist, Reach to Recovery Volunteer and the patient herself, whose goal was attainment of her own maximum recovery.

(Should you yourself require radiation therapy, do not

make the mistake Miss O'D. did—if you have questions about it, ask your physician for answers. He knows better than anyone. You may find the therapy boring, and on occasion fatiguing, but *do not fear it.* It is not painful. Pamper yourself with a nap afterward, if you're fatigued—resting when you are tired is especially important at this time.)

There in that little room Miss O'D. listened intently, nodding sometimes, saying little, but her fear seemed to be subsiding and her composure returning.

Then her surgeon, Dr. McK., came in, and I left the room to make my scheduled rounds of visiting other patients. The third of these visits had been completed when I was summoned to the phone. It was Dr. McK.: Our team effort, he said, had been rewarded; recovery for little Miss O'D. would be like that of any other mastectomy patient, and he had decided to withhold the psychiatric consultation for the present.

It has always seemed to me that a woman's demeanor and manner of dress signal to the world her inner spirit and character. For those of us who have had a mastectomy, this is doubly true. Do not, now, shun style or hide from fashion. This is the time for a fresh look at both, with making them work for you in mind. Carelessness in dress or indifference to smartness are quite inexcusable. You are the same person you have always been, and can become even better—so dress up to that concept. *It's a great boost to your femininity to wear the right clothes at the right time in the right place.*

Daytime and evening attire need pose no more of a problem for you now than it did prior to your operation. Many ready-made dresses will be perfect. Scarves and stoles may be worn with flair and distinction.

In wintertime, soft woolen clothing should get top priority in your wardrobe during those months immediately following your operation—it enhances your comfort besides being correct for the season.

In summer there is no reason whatsoever not to wear pretty dresses or bathing suits as you always have. Some may need building up a bit, or taking up at the shoulder.

In case of skin discoloration sometimes resulting from radiation, several cosmetic preparations are on the market. One of the best ones in my opinion is Covermark. This can be purchased in most drugstores or the cosmetics counters of department stores, or directly from the manufacturer. Oncc your doctor approves of your using them, it is simply a matter of selecting the waterproof shade closest in tone to the clear skin surrounding the discoloration. Of course, after your skin has been exposed to radiation it needs pampering, such as avoiding direct rays of sunlight for hours on end. Protect the areas that have received therapy by wearing a scarf or some other covering.

As to bedtime attire, whatever you are accustomed to wearing—pajamas or a nightgown—need not be changed at all, other than perhaps a minimal adjustment or two. Dress for bed with one fact firmly in mind: *There's no need to change anything because you yourself have not changed; you're the same person you've always been.* If the esthetics bother you, soft nylon net ruching formed into a full, roselike shape and sewn into your nightgown or pajamas will give the desired effect. It is sometimes more comfortable to sew a small, soft covering such as rubber or soft material over the gathered stitches.

If you feel it essential to wear a breast form to bed (and I, for one, do not) night bras are available at some stores.

Or you can make one yourself: Cut an old bra in half. Sew a firm piece of ribbon on the back end, bring the ribbon around to within 6 inches of the front center of the bra and sew a 6-inch length of elastic to the ribbon. Sew a hook on the end of the elastic and an eye on the front end of the bra, then hook the elastic to the bra. Either make a pocket for your prosthesis or sew it into the night bra. A 6-inch piece of elastic should be sewn in back of the remaining shoulder strap. These night bras should be loose and not interfere with your sleeping comfort. New lounge bras are available at very little cost. Soft and stretchy, one even has pockets on both sides that go up to the shoulder and enable you to use a filler if needed.

And finally, as to beach attire: A woman in San Francisco wrote, *"I can't possibly understand how you can wear a bathing suit. I have a deep scar which extends out to the upper part of my arm. I also had grafting done, so have a bad scar visible on my thigh."* Covermark solved her problem.

Another woman wrote, *"I love swimming but didn't go near the water last year because I'm on the hefty side, and need a large bra, 42 to be exact, and I don't know where to find a specially built bathing suit."*

If you happen to be on the large side and cannot find a suit long enough for you, buy a becoming *lined* sleeveless dress or use one of your own (or an unlined dress and attach a full slip), put the hem up to the desired length, and wear your own bra and form. Buy matching colored jersey panties. Wear two pairs. You'll find it works beautifully.

The right attire for bathing has been a major problem for many women—and it need not be a problem at all.

One of our Reach to Recovery Volunteers had a child who was four years old—the age for "Why?" questioning. After her mastectomy, the child began asking his mother why she would never go swimming with him. Eventually she ran out of excuses and came to us with the problem. A couple of hours spent in trying on bathing suits, and there was no longer any need for her to hide from her little son or anyone else on the beach.

If swimming has been one of your favorite pastimes, do not give it up after your operation. It is one of the best exercises for you. In all probability you will be able to wear your present swimsuit with very little alteration. Or, if a new one will provide a needed boost to your morale, some of the foremost designers include in their lines a wide range of styles suitable for women who have had mastectomies, styles in no visible way any different from those being worn by women who have not had this surgery: "Two-piece Mio with bolero top" . . . "tank suit with semi-boy leg" . . . "high-neck maillot with cut-out back" . . . "two-piece tunic top over pleated skirt" . . . "V-neck tunic and contrasting skirt" . . . "stretch nylon stripe terry jumpsuit" . . . "Mio jumpsuit with long sleeves and zipper front" . . . our yearly list of swimsuit styles goes on and on, changing as the fashions change, with styles as comfortable for you as they are flattering.

Insert your breast form in a pocket in your bathing suit, or wear a bra-and-form under the suit, or sew rubber forms securely into the suit. If your suit has a built-in bra and this is not comfortable, cut the back off one of your old bras and sew the front part into the suit, attaching it to the side seams. You can use the same type pocket that you use in your bras. If you prefer, you may sew a rubber form in the bathing suit or inside a pocket and leave it in the suit permanently.

If a bra is your preference, sew in five restraints to hold it in place; large lingerie straps will do. Attach one in the center front, one on each side at the seams, and one on each side of the zipper in back. The notions-and-trimmings counters in most department stores stock a tape which has snap fasteners set at regularly spaced intervals; this will serve the purpose. Or if you wish you can make your own.

If your breast form is rubber, remember when you come out of the pool or surf to squeeze the water out of it. This is easily managed, poolside or on a crowded beach—just use a towel to dry your face and while making a pretense of wiping your eyes press your prosthesis with your raised forearm. No one will be the wiser!

In the years since the Reach to Recovery Program was able to help Nelle W. to achieve a "natural look," her distinguished husband, Dr. W., has approved the Program for many of his patients.

It is encouraging that, thanks to the efforts of the American Cancer Society's Service and Rehabilitation Program, Dr. W. and other physicians today recognize that medical personnel are relieved of time-consuming activities not primarily medical in nature, through this rehabilitation service.

And to the patient—to you, yourself—when we of Reach to Recovery say, "You can dress as well as ever; you can present to the world an even better-groomed, smarter-looking You than before your operation," we are speaking truly, as always, woman to woman, out of similar experience.

VII

"Action Absorbs Anxiety"

IN 1913, when few cancer patients had any hope of cure, the American Society for the Control of Cancer (now the American Cancer Society) was founded as a voluntary health agency to fight this disease until it was conquered.

Today, almost sixty years later, *1,500,000 men, women and children in the United States who had cancer are alive and cured* of cancer. At this writing, more than 200,000 Americans will be saved from cancer in 1972, according to the American Cancer Society's own "Facts and Figures" data estimate.

From the day of its founding, the Society has crusaded in the fields of research, education, and service to the patient. To find an appropriate symbol for its crusade, a nationwide poster contest was sponsored. The design selected by the Society was a drawn sword, its blade flashing the spirit of the cancer control movement, its twin-serpent caduceus hilt emphasizing the medical and scientific aspects of the attack. Known as The Sword of Hope, it has come to reflect the image and identity of the ACS.

In 1928, when this sword symbol came into being, fewer than one patient in five was being saved.

Ten years later, it was one in four.

Today it is one in three—and on the way to becoming one in two.

The authoritative journal *Cancer Research,* partly supported by the American Cancer Society and official organ of the American Association for Cancer Research, states that there are definite "portents of victory": "The concept of a virus-cell symbiosis . . . is no longer only a hypothesis. . . . Immunizations for some forms of human cancers are not far away." The journal stresses the fact that several major forms of the disease can now be prevented. Surgery and radiation therapy are constantly being improved, and certain forms of cancers yield to chemical or hormone treatment. And what has long been emphasized by the ACS is reaffirmed in the journal, that "Early diagnosis, early effective treatment will always be necessary. The extension of preventive, therapeutic and rehabilitative facilities . . . remains our goal."

The Reach to Recovery Program is such a rehabilitative facility.

The Director of New York University's Institute for Rehabilitation, speaking at an American Cancer Society-sponsored meeting about rehabilitation's role in achieving maximum patient recovery, stated that the greatest antidote in the world for acute postoperative depression is activity. His phrase was "Action Absorbs Anxiety."

For women who have had a mastectomy, indeed thank God for action which can absorb anxiety!

When my children were small, their father once asked them to sit down, think very carefully, and make a list of what they were most thankful to God for. Here is what my son, age seven at the time, wrote: "I thank God for sunshine after rainy days in spring. And for my dog Toby. For my friend Dean. For the humming birds. Trees to climb. And things to do."

Things to do—for all its innocence, this was wisdom. The value of comprehensive action following a mastectomy cannot be overemphasized. It is the keystone of the entire Reach to Recovery Program. Within three months after my release from the hospital, I was swimming and playing golf, entertaining at home and being entertained in the homes of friends. I was driving my car—and I didn't have power steering, either! It was not easy. Sometimes it hurt, but each small victory over physical handicap gave a boost to my morale and my entire attitude.

It seems to me that *attitude* is at the core of personality. It is what makes a person tick, what makes us what we are. To define it simply as a state of mind is not enough. *Attitude is that state of emotional readiness for experience* which, at its best, can make anything possible for us.

When I first met her, Julie T. was emotionally ready for any experience that might come her way. A member of the graduating class at the first school of nursing where I spoke about the Reach to Recovery Program, Julie was then a bride of six months, and just pregnant. Her attitude was buoyant, positive, idealistic, brimming with the most glowing plans for the future. Her personality fairly sparkled, making her a thoroughly delightful person to know. Following her graduation we kept in touch via letters, cards exchanged at Christmas, and lunches whenever I was in Richmond, where Julie worked.

But then, three months into pregnancy, Julie suffered a miscarriage. Over the next five years, she miscarried four times. Her doctor assured her that she could still, with prudence, carry a baby to term. But Julie's personality had begun to change. She no longer wanted a baby. Children of any age, in or out of the hospital, set her nerves on edge. So did anyone who crossed her in any way. Her popularity in the hospital waned. Friends drifted away. Her marriage started to go downhill. Her letters took on a tone of irritability and complaint about her husband who was unreasonable, her co-workers who were untrustworthy, her supervisor who "had it in for her," the patients who were ill-tempered malingerers and causing her work to suffer. Her conversation, on the occasions when we were together, was self-centered and full of her troubles—none of which, to hear Julie tell them, were due to Julie's own shortcomings.

It was scarcely a surprise when a letter came, finally, saying that her marriage was ending in a divorce and Julie was resigning from the hospital staff.

My reply to that letter was worded most carefully. Most of it dwelt on the high cost of a negative attitude. It was never answered. No card arrived from Julie the following Christmas. On my next trip to Richmond, I tried to reach her by phone and was told she had left the city. And gone where? No one knew, and no one seemed to care much.

It was years before I heard from Julie again. An article of mine appeared in *McCall's* and she wrote saying she had read it. She had been living in the Midwest with the older sister who had raised her—and shortly after leaving Richmond she had undergone a mastectomy.

"Sister was wonderfully considerate when I came home from the hospital," Julie wrote, "and I just lay around soaking up attention. Having a sympathetic audience, I moaned and groaned and felt terribly sorry for myself. For weeks I just wallowed in depression." Then, due to failing health, the older sister had gone into a nursing home. "Without her, I of necessity had to make beds, vacuum floors, wash dishes, do the marketing. I had no one to complain to, and no time for complaining. In about one week I was completely cured, both physically and mentally. You said something in a letter a long time ago on the advantages of a positive attitude. How true that is!

"As far as I'm concerned," Julie added, "the secret of keeping one's sanity after this operation is Work!"

The letter's tone was certainly not that of the sparkling young woman I remembered from long ago. But it was not that of the whining defeatist woman, either. This was a new Julie, with a new attitude—and a new life because of it: "I have married again," she concluded, "and my marriage is as close to perfection as a marriage can be. Neither of us ever thinks at all about the operation."

The antidote for depression for her had surely been action. And the prelude to action was that state of emotional readiness, a positive attitude.

The sooner your own attitude spurs a return to activity, the better.

Your physician is the one to say when "soon" will be. But once he approves, you should waste no time getting back into the mainstream of living.

Of course do not overdo. Do not fatigue yourself. But do not, in the process of being active, neglect the following important attentions to the hand and arm on the side of your operation.

Any skin area which has received X-ray therapy should also be protected from overexposure to the sun.

These precautions are necessary because it is so important that you not run the risk of infection. But they are not an

Please read these points carefully and think about how they apply to your way of life and your daily activities.

1. When working around the house, take care to avoid burns and other injuries.
2. When sewing, use a thimble to protect the end of your finger.
3. When gardening, wear strong work gloves to guard against scratches and cuts.
4. When doing dishes or laundry, avoid maceration of the skin from prolonged immersion in water.
5. When doing housework, don't move heavy furniture or lift heavy objects—have someone help you.
6. When giving yourself a manicure, be careful not to cut the cuticle. Use a lanolin-base lotion to keep the cuticle soft.
7. When out in the sun, cover your arm with a light scarf or handkerchief; swelling may occur from too much sunburn, so take care to avoid it.
8. No blood samples for tests should be taken from your affected arm, nor should it be vaccinated or receive injections. Use the other arm for having blood pressure taken.

excuse to delay a return to your normal activity. How you were active before your operation is how you should be active now.

If you drove a car before, start driving again.

If you played tennis or golf, play again.

If you were working at a career, go to work at it again.

If you enjoyed dancing, or going to the theater, or entertaining friends and being entertained by them, begin to enjoy all those activities again.

And do what you do—driving, playing, working, enjoying—without emotional fanfare. No one is favored by reminders of your operation, but no one is comfortable with exaggerated reticence about it, either. Since it is very much on your mind, confiding in friends is a perfectly natural thing to do, provided your confidence is welcomed and placed in the right people.

Any friend who is genuinely interested and genuinely trying to be helpful should receive your trust and confidence. By all means accept that help. Appreciate that interest. But do not exploit either.

Cultivate the attitude that your operation is an event of the past. Your former routine of living was interrupted by it, but now it's over, so life goes on as usual. Think that, believe it, and life *will* go on as usual—with every likelihood of becoming even better.

And in the sweetness of friendship let there be laughter, and the sharing of pleasures.
For in the dew of little things the heart finds its morning and is refreshed.

—KAHLIL GIBRAN, *The Prophet*

People do need people. Sociability is vital to our well-being and development.

Psychologists tell us it is the personal relationships in life which create the individual—the Self. No one is born with a personality. That is shaped for us, stretched and tempered, every day of our lives by every other personality with whom we come in contact.

And if for any reason we deny ourselves this contact with others, we are inviting trouble.

"The source of all the basic anxieties in human nature," Liebman says, "is a feeling of being alone and helpless in a hostile world." He goes on to stress the importance of building a bridge of fellowship "between ourselves and . . . the friend, the co-worker." According to Norman Vincent Peale, it is worth a lifetime's effort to perfect "your great capacities for friendliness . . . personal relationships are vitally important to successful living."

For the outgoing woman who is relaxed and confident with people, sociability will be little or no problem following a mastectomy. That is one less obstacle for her to surmount on the road to recovery.

But not everyone is outgoing. Not everyone is relaxed and confident with people. There are those who are retiring and shy, reticent by nature. There are those who have become sparing in their trust, and wary about their confidants. If you happen to be such a person, now is the time to make an effort to change. See yourself not as a solitary individual, independent and isolated from everyone else, but as one part of a complex of relationships with others.

See yourself like that—nurture that attitude—and the rewards in speeding your recovery and expanding your enjoyment of life will, I promise you, more than repay the effort.

This was reaffirmed for me when, prior to attending a symposium on rehabilitation, I spent a weekend with friends at their cottage in Maine. Across the lake was a sprawling white frame house flanked by a weathered barn and several neat shedlike structures. Set on an expanse of green lawn sloping down to the water's edge, it had a lovely old-homestead look, like something out of a Currier & Ives print.

My hostess identified it as one of the numerous summer resorts in the area.

"By the way," her husband said, "they'll be square dancing over there tonight. How about dropping in to watch the fun?"

The public was invited to this once-a-week entertainment at the resort, and when we arrived the big barn was already crowded. A fiddler was scraping away at "Cindy," a hoarse-voiced caller was clutching a hand mike, and three sets of four couples were allemande-ing gaily, more or less in time with the music and the calls. Spectators outnumbered dancers. We started around the room searching for seats on one of the benches along the wall.

"Now do-si—the ladies—do," the caller sang. "With a couple of gents you ought to know, just one more change and there's your beau!"

My hostess indicated a plump woman in one of the formations who was walking lightly through the "do-si-do." Judging from the brightness of her smile, no one in the place was having a happier time, or enjoying herself more.

"Would you believe she's the town wallflower?" my friend whispered.

"Was," her husband corrected. "Ex-wallflower. Look."

"Balance four in the middle of the floor," the caller sang. "Swing your honey like swinging on a gate, swing her round till she yells 'Wait!' "

The woman, who looked to be in her mid-thirties, was anything but a wallflower. Her exuberance was setting the mood for her partner and the other couples in the set. No quadrille on the floor was livelier.

"Five weeks ago," my friend murmured, "Maggie was on the operating table." I looked at her quickly. She nodded. "A radical mastectomy. Five weeks ago. Imagine. She wants so much to meet you."

During the rest of the evening, whenever Maggie sat out a dance (which wasn't often) she came over to chat. Before her operation, she said, she had weighed two hundred and thirty-nine pounds. As "the fat girl" in town, she had not only been a wallflower in and out of high school but felt herself an object of ridicule among her peers. No boys dated her, and most girls found her company a burden. "It was a sort of vicious circle," Maggie told me wryly. "The more they thought I was a bore, the more boring I actually was." The time came when, tired of feeling unwanted and unwelcomed, she broke off what few friendships she had made, stopped going to Grange meetings and church socials—shut herself away from social contacts altogether—and was well on the way to becoming the town eccentric before she was forty.

Then she had discovered she must undergo a mastectomy.

"That," Maggie said earnestly, "just turned my life right around. It pointed me in a whole new direction."

It most certainly had, judging from appearances that evening.

"I don't mean the operation itself." She explained that in order to take her mind off the pending surgery she had started to clean house one day, "top to bottom." In a second-floor closet she came across a dusty stack of old magazines. One was a 1954 issue of *Coronet,* containing an article of mine titled "After Breast Surgery."

"It gave me hope," Maggie said, "that I could come through it like you did. I knew then exactly what I had to do to help myself—change my attitude, believe in myself, have faith in other people, live life instead of hiding from it."

A ruggedly handsome man came up to us. "It's 'Grand

Square,' Maggie, with all the trimmings," he said.

"In a minute, Hank." She waved him away, and stood up. "I truly do believe," Maggie said, "that that article was a blueprint for my future. And it had been up in that closet, gathering dust, for twelve years."

Quadrilles were forming out on the floor. Her handsome partner was beckoning impatiently. Maggie held out her hand and I stood up to take it.

"One thing's for sure," Maggie said, "it was no happenstance. It was there when I needed it." The bright smile was back, but her eyes held tears, too. "That blueprint for my future was kept there for me all those years by my Higher Power. . . ."

Watching her take her place with the others, I thought of that sound counsel, *Build a bridge to fellowship. . . . Perfect your capacities for friendliness. . . .* That was what Maggie was doing, all right, and that was why what she called her blueprint for her future was going to build her a good life.

It was once widely believed that we, as individuals, are helpless to control our lot in life.

Nowadays psychologists tell us that anyone, by developing her capacities to fulfill her own potential, can make of her life what she will.

The first step in doing this is to understand, and believe, that within each of us there are these wonderful capacities, waiting to be tapped.

No one ever tapped them better than Mrs. P.Z.'s mother, a woman who did not even accord the word "helpless" a place in her vocabulary.

As her daughter described her in a letter to Reach to Recovery, this woman was a dramatic example of how to make use of life instead of permitting life to use you.

"My mother had a mastectomy twenty-one years ago," Mrs. P.Z. wrote. "At the time she was employed in a hat factory where she used her hands and arms constantly. She returned to her job, and did all her own housework and baked her own bread besides, which requires a lot of motion." A few years later, Mrs. P.Z.'s sister became sickly, so "She moved in with my mother and father. At the same time my father had his leg amputated." At this point, Mrs. P.Z.'s mother left her job, took over the care of her husband and sickly daughter, continued to do her own housework and marketing, "and washed and ironed for seven people.

"Now she is seventy-two," the letter continued, "and people say she is the friendliest person, always ready with a smile. She never looked for sympathy and just resumed her life as if she never had an operation. At times her arm would swell but she never stopped doing anything. She has always been cheerful and people like having her around them."

Although I never met this remarkable woman, some years later I did meet Mrs. P.Z. herself, at one of our open forums, and had an opportunity to thank her in person for that letter.

"Well," she said, "I thought you might come across some patients who were discouraged. I wanted them to know they will be able to do anything they set their minds to, if they are just determined like my mother was."

And I remember thinking that being determined was only part of it. That woman made the most of a great capacity for friendliness, too. She seemed to know instinctively how vital sociability was to her well-being.

If sociability is difficult for you—and for many women it is, after this operation—these six suggestions should make it a bit easier, and your recovery a bit more rapid:

1. Remind yourself, every day, that everyone you meet is a potential enrichment of your own personality. Turn your thoughts outward toward them, instead of inward toward yourself.

2. Practice listening sympathetically to others' problems rather than talking about your own. There is an art to being a good listener, and it is well worth learning.

3. Tell yourself that "So-and-so is really unique," then search out that uniqueness. You will find it if you look for it, because it is there, in each of us.

4. Let people know you trust them and want their friendship. Applaud their achievements as you'd like them to applaud your own.

5. Make yourself a more interesting person by keeping up with what is going on in the world. Form opinions about many things, but try to be opinionated about nothing.

6. Keep in mind that "action absorbs anxiety," and that a positive attitude is the prelude to action, and the key to sociability.

VIII

Love Yourself to Enjoy Life

ONE OF MY YOUNG FRIENDS had an aunt with what the niece termed "a weird hangup"—she refused to refer to any living thing as an "it." Thus, to this lady a dandelion was "he," as was an oak tree or any goldfish more than three inches in length; water-lilies and buttercups, on the other hand, would be called "she." Quite frankly, I suspected my young friend of making this up—until the day her aunt saw my prize cyclamen in bloom and exclaimed, "She loves herself! How nice of her to show it."

House plants have always been my particular delight. They crowd my home and my office—coleus, peperomias, nephthytis, pandanus, Whittington ferns, Christmas cactus, African violets, dieffenbachias, Rex begonias. Tending them at day's end is like relaxing in the undemanding company of old friends.

When the seven-year-old cyclamen blooms in midwinter, "she" bears as many as thirty flowers at one time. Florists tell me it is unusual, without benefit of a greenhouse, to keep these plants from year to year and bring them into bloom. They credit a "green thumb." But I rather like that other explanation—"She loves herself"—which is to say, *she fulfills herself.*

All forms of life seek self-fulfillment. As human beings, it is surely vital to our inner peace.

And when a woman has undergone a mastectomy, this inner peace, or "self-love," is essential to her maximum recovery. Narcissism (psychology's term for self-centered pampering and indulgence) should not be confused with proper self-love—it is not the same thing at all. "Love yourself to enjoy life" simply means *respect yourself enough to make the most of life.*

The one great gift—indeed the only lifetime gift—which has been bestowed by God upon every woman is herself. Surely we owe it to Him not to demean or belittle His gift. Yet each time we underestimate our self we *do* demean it. Each time we see only our faults, while minimizing our assets, we *are* belittling it.

And when we do that, it is we who are the losers—as Marion B. had been a loser most of her life.

Marion was a supervisor of social workers in Brooklyn. In the course of my work I had come to know her rather well. Far from ever showing any proper self-love, Marion did not seem to like herself at all. One of the hospital administrators labeled her a chronic complainer, and with reason: For Marion, nothing, ever, was satisfactory, and what she was mostly dissatisfied with was herself: She should have handled the X Case better; or, Why wasn't she quicker to grasp Y's problem? or, If only she had been more patient with Z! She had the lowest possible opinion of herself, yet the fact was she did her work well and worked very hard. The trouble was, "duty" amounted to a fetish with her, and the exalted standards she set for herself to "measure up" were so far beyond her capacities that nothing Marion did ever satisfied Marion.

When she underwent a mastectomy and asked to see me some days after the operation, I expected to encounter post-operative self-loathing of the most acute sort.

Her room was full of flowers—surprisingly, because this woman had never seemed to have many friends. Flowering plants and vases of cut flowers were on the bureau and lined up along the window sill. Get-well cards rimmed the mirror above the bureau. Marion was sitting up in bed, talking on the phone. She greeted me with a smile and a half-wave—using her hand on the side of the operation, which had apparently already benefited from exercising. Her voice, as she thanked someone on the phone for her thoughtfulness, was warm and relaxed, and with none of its usual sharp edge of fretful discontent.

It was not at all what I'd expected, and my astonishment must have shown as Marion put down the phone.

"When they started coming," she said, indicating the cards and flowers, "I told the nurses somebody'd goofed, they couldn't all be for me. But it turned out they were for me. Isn't it wonderful?"

What was even more wonderful was Marion's new attitude, and I said so.

She nodded gravely. For the first few days after surgery, she said, she had wished herself dead. "It sickened me to think what I'd have to look at in the mirror for the rest of my life." She hated God for letting this happen to her, she hated the doctor for finding the lump in her breast and the surgeon for performing the operation. Most of all she hated herself for being, as she put it, "not fit even to be called a woman any more."

Then the mail began bringing get-well cards. The florists

began delivering flowers and plants. "I couldn't believe what was happening. I said to myself, who would bother? Who cares this much about me?"

A few of the senders' names she recognized—her sister, a cousin, the co-workers on her service. Most, though, were names only vaguely familiar. "But all of a sudden it hit me. 'The Jodine Family,' sure, I worked out a place for them to stay after they'd been evicted from their apartment. And 'Clara Meade,' I helped reconcile her with her husband. 'Mr. and Mrs. Canfield,' I've been counseling their runaway daughter." One by one, people she had helped and was still helping were saying "Thanks. Get well. You're needed."

Marion reached for a tissue and blew her nose.

"I look around this room now," she said, "and I think, 'My girl, you have been selling yourself short. If you're okay with this many folks, be at least a little bit okay with yourself.'" Her eyes brimmed and she looked quickly away. "For the first time in my life I don't feel inadequate. I don't feel that I'm a flop. It sounds funny to put it into words, but I've begun to like myself—" She hesitated, and her gaze came back to meet mine. "That is the strangest sensation," she said softly. "I mean, liking myself. It's as if I'm more of a whole person, now, than I have ever been before."

Three short weeks later, when I saw Marion B. back at her desk, I recalled what she'd said that day: *Liking myself . . . I'm more of a whole person than I have ever been before.*

Proper esteem of self, psychologists tell us, is at the very core of maturity. It is also, surely, at the heart of genuine femininity. A woman must be at peace with herself in order to be at peace with her environment—whether that is a career or the home, as a wife and mother.

"Self-love," Voltaire wrote, "is the instrument of our preservation."

On a TV broadcast about the drug culture, an ex-addict was filmed saying, "It's when you know you're Somebody that you don't need a fix."

After four years in a Communist prison camp, an American major on his release told newsmen, "None of my men broke. None of my men defected. Because none of us forgot who we are, or what we are."

Self-love—the instrument of our preservation. And its opposite is the seed which germinates our destruction: self-hate—whose fruit is a wasting sense of personal inferiority. Time and again, following a woman's mastectomy, I have seen the damage done to her physical and mental well-being by an unreasoning hatred of self.

When I was in Israel, I saw such hatred come very close to destroying one woman.

My path crossed Mrs. T.Y.'s some years ago, after I'd spent a long day working with a group at Hadassah Hospital in Jerusalem. The following morning, while my companions were touring the hospital, I used the time before we must catch our bus back to Tel-Aviv to go to the Chapel for a glimpse of the famous Chagall murals there.

The Chapel, which is only a few steps from the hospital, was empty. Wooden benches stood at opposite ends of the room, and I chose a seat where I could best appreciate the magnificent paintings.

Presently, two women entered and, ignoring the murals, sat on one of the benches across the Chapel.

The taller of the two was a physiotherapist I had met on the previous evening. Her companion had a stolid, rawboned look of hard toil about her. Hunched forward on the bench, feet planted far apart, elbows on knees, big-knuckled hands methodically ripping to shreds a page from a newspaper, she appeared oblivious to what the therapist was saying to her.

My time was running out. To reach the exit it was necessary to pass within a few feet of the women, and someone spoke my name.

It was the therapist. She introduced her companion as Mrs. T.Y., just arrived from a kibbutz far to the north in the region of the Dan, where the borders of Israel touch Syria. The woman herself did not look up or speak. The therapist explained that the tedious journey from the kibbutz to Jerusalem had been undertaken to learn, firsthand, about the Reach to Recovery Program: Mrs. T.Y. had had a mastectomy some months before and was in need of help. A newspaper publicizing the lecture, strewn now in bits and pieces across the floor, testified to her feelings on having discovered her journey had been for nothing, that she had arrived a day too late to benefit from the lecture.

"I brought her into the Chapel to quiet her," the therapist said. "I've been repeating some of what you told our group last evening, but she came all this distance to hear it from you, personally. Really, when I glanced up and saw that you were still here, I couldn't believe my eyes."

For the first time, Mrs. T.Y. spoke. "I am a stupid fool," she said. Her voice was harsh, almost guttural. "All I do, ever, is make stupid mistakes." Her heavy shoulders lifted in an impatient, writhing shrug.

"She blames herself," the therapist said, "for missing bus connections on the way here."

"Nothing comes out good for me," Mrs. T.Y. said. "Why? Because I don't deserve that it should, that is why." She sounded angry, bitter, thoroughly disgusted with herself.

I glanced at my watch. Another two minutes, and I would be missing my own bus connections.

A thought occurred to me: Having come so far to get help, suppose Mrs. T.Y. came a little farther, to Tel-Aviv, with me? "We can talk on the bus," I suggested, "and when we get to my hotel there, I'll work with you." Unless, that is, time was a factor for her? Was she in a hurry to return to her home?

"Before I return to my home," Mrs. T.Y. said flatly, "I would kill myself."

And she meant precisely that, as I learned on the bus a few moments later. Here was a woman despising herself enough to wish to destroy herself. Her recent breast surgery had fueled that wish—"Why should my husband want to live with me now?"—and so had a persistent lymphedema which left her unable to fulfill her obligations to the kibbutz. But she had had a sense of abject inferiority long before she had a mastectomy, and the roots of her self-hate spread in many directions through her personality.

Her husband, for example, was a man she knew to be her intellectual superior, and in fifteen years of marriage she had fallen so far off his pace that she was convinced they no longer shared any interests in common. She felt isolated, alone, unloved, the object of her man's disdain, the butt of his friends' ridicule. And when she said that two abortions early in life had left her unable to bear children, it was clear that guilt over that was yet another ego-destroying reminder of her unworthiness as a wife and a woman.

We talked quietly, in the rear of the bus, all the way to Tel-Aviv. For the most part, Mrs. T.Y. did the talking while I tried to listen sympathetically.

But sympathy for such self-contempt does not come easily.

Several times I came close to retorting, If you are an inferior person it is because you have branded yourself inferior—and for no other reason. I almost said, The only shame you have a right to feel is over your shabby treatment of yourself. No one else, I wanted to tell her, husband and friends included, could spare the time to lavish on you the disdain and ridicule which you've lavished on yourself.

"A stupid fool" had been this woman's first words about herself—and somehow she must be made to understand, for her own sake, that a stupid fool is her own worst enemy. But could she be made to understand that, without taking offense? The last thing I wanted to do was hurt her more than she had already hurt herself. We would work together, as I had promised, when we got to Tel-Aviv—but her endless listings of personal shortcomings without mention of a single virtue to offset them had me wondering, frankly, whether it would be worth the effort.

The next day, Mrs. T.Y.'s introduction to the Reach to Recovery Program was rigorous and exacting. Three strenuous work sessions were crammed into the next forty-eight hours—and proved to be very much worth the effort. Mrs. T.Y.'s progress was remarkable—as exercises helped the lymphedema a little, her arm regained a bit more mobility, and thanks to a new prosthesis, properly fitted, there was a marked improvement in her appearance.

But "stupid fool" and "inferior" still had to be erased from her thinking, by helping her to find peace within herself so she could be at peace with her environment, and that would take time, which by then was all but gone: my schedule called for leaving Tel-Aviv that weekend. After our third work session together, there would be no opportunity to see

Mrs. T.Y. again before moving on to Haifa, where my last lecture in Israel was to be given.

On my tours abroad, the last few hours tend to telescope—suddenly there is too much to do and too little time left for doing it. Attendance at the lecture in Haifa doubled the expected turnout; the two hours allotted for it stretched to four; farewells were protracted, and delaying. It was a scant five minutes before departure time when I arrived, somewhat breathless, at the airport.

Waiting at the departure gate was Mrs. T.Y.

She had followed me from Tel-Aviv to Haifa just to say goodbye. There was no time to express how deeply that touched me. Our paths had crossed so briefly, yet we had become friends. Neither of us would soon forget the other.

Where was she going from here?

Home, she said. Her eyes were bright. She did not say that she had found inner peace. She did not mention her husband, or her obligations to the kibbutz. What she said was, "I am not ashamed now. So, maybe, things will be different."

Boarding my plane, I looked back to wave. Mrs. T.Y. also was waving. *I am not ashamed,* she had said. Yes, I thought, things will be different for her now.

As the Society's *Annual Report* says, "International co-operation in cancer control is as dynamic as the changing world map!"

Cooperation between the American Cancer Society and cancer societies in other countries is worldwide and ever expanding. For example, American Cancer Society guidance helped organize societies in Indonesia and in the African Republic of Zambia, and the fact that the former was founded by one of the participants in a special ACS graduate course for physicians of the Far East and Oceania is a source of particular pride to us. The ACS special graduate course for Latin American physicians was followed up by similarly sponsored postgraduate courses in Buenos Aires, Argentina, and in Lima, Peru, with distinguished faculty members from the United States working with specialists in both areas to present programs adapting new techniques to local facilities and conditions. In Cali, Colombia, the Society's assistance was vital in launching a cancer-control program whose results will be of worldwide interest. Key people from Yugoslavia and Iceland have been served by a special ACS training course. Our Society hosted the Tenth International Cancer Congress, in Houston, at which more than six thousand men and women representing 72 nations came together in a spirit of international exchange to share thoughts on the cancer battle. The Society helps support the International Union Against Cancer (UICC), and in turn this Geneva-based organization administers one of the most important ACS programs, the American Cancer Society–Eleanor Roosevelt International Cancer Fellowships.

"Hate yourself, and you'll judge yourself unfairly," warns Dr. Liebman. "Beware a feeling of inferiority, and attributing to others abilities and powers which they don't possess. Beneath their lacquer of poise and assurance, they too bear scars of doubts and failure."

The wise woman will heed this warning. And when she has had a mastectomy, she will know better than to tolerate even for a moment any feeling of inferiority.

A Reach to Recovery Volunteer reported on such a patient, a woman who had never in all her life been inside a hospital until, within a space of thirteen months, she underwent five operations. As she put it to the Volunteer, "If that wouldn't turn you sour on yourself, I'd like to know. But it hasn't got me down and I don't intend to let it." The nurses appreciated this woman's spirit, and brought in other patients so she might cheer them up. "They ask me how I can be so light-hearted. My answer is, 'Smile and the world smiles with you—weep and you weep alone.' They ask me what I have to smile about. I tell them, 'Every day I live, I'm that much more of a person than I was the day before.' "

Another such spirited woman wrote that "The greatest change in me since my operation is one of mental attitude and emotional outlook. Because tomorrow was a big question mark for me not long ago, today has become very precious. I am learning to live in the present, casting off those anxieties about the future which weigh so heavily on many women."

Hubert Benoit, in his unique dialogues entitled *The Many Faces of Love,* has offered sound advice to the woman who might feel, ever, for any reason, inferior. "Whenever you suffer from the idea," M. Benoit wrote, "dispel the thought by remembering your matchless aptitude—as a woman—for devotion, all the exquisite delicacy and indomitable strength you can bring to the care of the one you love."

Every mature woman possesses this God-given aptitude. Surgery cannot excise it. No operation can diminish it. Only the woman herself—you, yourself—can do that. You alone can void the essence of your own femininity by yielding to the idea that you are, because of your operation, somehow inferior.

Remember, *Self-love is the instrument of our preservation,* and remember at the same time a further admonition of M. Benoit's that *A feeling of humiliation within a woman may destroy her self-love.*

Several years ago that feeling of humiliation—so wrong, so foolish!—almost shattered the careers, the hopes and the happiness of two extraordinarily fine people from "Down Under."

Not yet having been to Australia or New Zealand at the time, I got to know Art and Laurie without our ever actually having met. Through a foreign exchange graduate nurse who knew them both—and especially thanks to Art himself—I came to know their story and to play a small but rather vital part in it.

Art had been born and raised in Tasmania, Laurie in New South Wales, and they had come together in Melbourne, where he was a mining engineer and she was a nurse. They became engaged and set a wedding date six months hence, by which time Art would have completed a field assignment at a mining camp in New Zealand. It would be a second marriage for them both. Art was in his early fifties, Laurie a year or two younger—but for all the maturity of their years their romance had a youthful exuberance that would have done credit to a pair of twenty-year-olds.

Two months after leaving Laurie in Melbourne and arriving at the mining camp in New Zealand, Art received a letter from her which stunned him.

Writing from the hospital, Laurie told him that she had undergone a mastectomy. She could not, she wrote, ask Art to spend the rest of his life with a woman who was, in her words, "not all there." So she was breaking off their engagement.

Art was frantic. He telephoned Laurie from the camp that

night. The connection was poor, so that neither heard the other clearly; the crackling on the line was a reminder of the many miles separating them. Laurie heard Art saying that her operation could not possibly affect his love for her. Art heard Laurie saying she loved him too much to tie him down to a cripple. He pleaded that she was the only woman he would ever love. She sobbed that some day he would find someone else—"A *complete* woman. So goodbye, Art."

The next mail to Melbourne carried a letter from Art begging Laurie to reconsider. The next mail from Melbourne carried Laurie's engagement ring, returned to Art. He tried to arrange for a leave of absence from the camp, to go and plead his case in person. He was told that a leave could not be arranged at that time. He tried to borrow money to fly to Melbourne without leave. Payday being three days off, no one had money to lend.

In his bitter frustration, Art confided his anguish to the infirmary's physician, Dr. F., and his wife Janet.

As a foreign exchange graduate nurse, Janet F. had spent a year on the staff of a large Manhattan hospital, where she attended one of my lectures. She recalled the stress placed by Reach to Recovery upon a patient's realizing that she is still very much "all there" after breast surgery—*You are the same person today as you were yesterday, and probably are safer, healthier, and better able to face the challenge of an even more rewarding tomorrow*—that phrase in particular Janet remembered reading in our *Reach to Recovery Manual,* and somewhere in her belongings she was sure that she still had a copy of that *Manual.* . . .

The airmail special delivery letter that came to Reach to Recovery with a New Zealand postmark was memorable. For one thing, it arrived on a birthday which was to be, for me, very special indeed. For another, its wording was so moving, with no attempt to mask a man's heartbreak: "If I could just go to her and be married, but that is impossible. . . . You see, it's a matter of setting her thinking straight about herself. . . . Right now, she hates herself and she thinks I would, too. . . . She talks about not being 'all there,' well, she will always be 'all there' for me, more than any other woman, but I can't make her understand that. . . . Hearing from somebody like yourself, who has come through this thing, might give her heart. . . . Please help her . . . please help us both."

Three hours after reading that letter, and already thirty minutes late for the birthday party planned by my family I was at the post office dropping two envelopes into a mail chute. One contained a brief note to Art, promising to do our best to be of help. The other contained a letter to Laurie, a long letter, very carefully worded to say, in effect, "Don't be a loser, my dear. Be good to yourself, and life will be so richly rewarding for you."

Had I guessed the surprise that was in store for me that evening, I should have been even more expansive on the subject of life's rewards.

Gifts had been unwrapped and exclaimed over, candles on a cake had been wished upon and puffed out, light-hearted toasts had been proposed and drunk, when suddenly a hush fell on the room. All eyes were on my brother-in-law, David Chase, who got slowly to his feet. I could sense an air of expectancy. And excitement. Everyone else seemed to know what was coming, but no one's face gave me a clue to what it might be.

"Thirteen years," David began, "is a long time to use an apartment to both live in and carry on a crusade. We've decided it has been long enough. We've decided that Reach to Recovery rates its own office, now."

He motioned to my son-in-law, Lee Gray, who winked at me and handed my brother-in-law a slim white envelope.

"It is a fact of life," David went on, "that office space in this city comes high. It is also a fact of life that one commodity Reach to Recovery lacks is funds. We talked the problem over with our partners, and they came up with a solution, this special gift to you."

He handed me the envelope.

My hands were shaking so I could scarcely open it. Inside was a plain white card. On the card were written breathtaking words: "Each year, for the next three years, Terese Lasser and Reach to Recovery will receive the sum of $10,000. Happy birthday from J. K. Lasser & Company."

It was one of those milestones which are so precious as to be remembered always.

There had been other milestones before: the initial publication of the *Manual,* for instance. And the generosity of anonymous donors, as well as those who would never accept payment for their help to the Program. The gift of $5,000 for three years from the Damon Runyon Fund was surely another. So was each hospital that accepted our Program. And each new group of Volunteers that was formed. Milestones all, precious all.

But this—coming as it did on my birthday, and from whom it came—well, it was as though, once again, my husband was at my side, telling me, "We all believe in you, so here is something to grow on."

To express heartfelt gratitude is such an art, and so often we do it inadequately . . .

My two friends "Down Under," by the way, did it very

well. The first holiday greeting I received the next year came from Melbourne, Australia. It was imprinted "Laurie and Arthur Barlow." And beneath the imprinting, in a firm feminine hand, was written, "God Bless, God Bless."

IX

"To Do Unto Others"

A NATIONWIDE Gallup study conducted for the American Cancer Society showed, among other findings, that nine out of ten women had heard of breast self-examination (Chapter IV) and that about half of these had done the examination at some time. However, only one woman in seven did so at the recommended monthly intervals.

Stressing the life-saving potential of early detection, the ACS urges every woman to

> **KNOW**
>
> **Cancer's Warning Signals!**
>
> **C**hange in bowel or bladder habits
>
> **A** sore that does not heal
>
> **U**nusual bleeding or discharge
>
> **T**hickening or lump in breast or elsewhere
>
> **I**ndigestion or difficulty in swallowing
>
> **O**bvious change in wart or mole
>
> **N**agging cough or hoarseness

If you have a warning signal, see your doctor.

A well-publicized breast cancer program conducted by the New York City Division of the Society brought a response of 1,300 letters and 2,000 telephone calls for information. This is just a single example of the effectiveness of the volunteer power on which every unit or division of the American Cancer Society primarily functions. An organization of more than two million Americans united to conquer cancer, the Society through its Volunteers brings information about every aspect of cancer control to the attention of men and women in every part of the country.

Of course I am very much aware of the help of the loyal and wonderful Volunteers who joined the Reach to Recovery program beginning with its early days and continuing through the years when we were "on our own." Many of those dedicated Volunteers continue to be active since our merger with the American Cancer Society in 1969. In addition, the Society has brought many new Volunteers into the Reach to Recovery Program. At this writing there are more than 3,000 trained Volunteers in about 1,500 hospitals in every part of the United States.

The heartbeat of Reach to Recovery, from the Volunteer point of view, is the desire of women who have been through the experience of a mastectomy, and triumphed over it, to help other women achieve their maximum recovery after this operation. For many women, it is a way of saying "Thank you" for their own recovery, and a way of doing something truly meaningful for others.

Some of my early letters from Volunteers bring this out. Mrs. Nora D. wrote me from Pasadena, California: "I underwent to mastectomy, survived, and returned home to live a perfectly normal life. Then I began to wonder about other women facing this same operation, and what I could do to ease their fears and help them fight and win." From Jacksonville, Illinois, Mrs. S.S.L. wrote, "I only wish I had had someone to come and talk to me when I was in the hospital. That is why I am writing. May I be of help?" From Miss L.V., of Miami, "I would love to help, I can't think of anything in this world I would rather do." And from I.R., in Detroit, "I'm sixty-seven and I'm not ready to be put on the shelf yet. I know I can help others to make the recovery I've made, if you will just tell me how." . . . These excerpts are from only a few of the letters written to me even before there was a formal Reach to Recovery Program, when I was struggling to get acceptance for the idea and to launch such a service.

Finally, when the idea had become a reality and spread from state to state and into many foreign countries, discussions began between officials of the American Cancer Society and myself about Reach to Recovery becoming a part of the Society's service-to-patients program, reflecting the Society's expanding concern for rehabilitation of all cancer patients. Early in 1969, the Board of Directors of the American Cancer Society approved a recommendation made by the Service Subcommittee on Rehabilitation of the Mastectomy Patient, which urged in part: "That the Society assume an active role [in this area of rehabilitation of the mastectomy patient] and that the first step be the incorporation of the 'Reach to Recovery' Program of Mrs. Terese Lasser into the Service Program as a commitment of the National Service Program."

It was a source of great satisfaction for all of us at Reach to Recovery to be able to bring to this forward-looking merger a budget surplus of $100,000 to contribute to the American Cancer Society's fight against cancer.

I became part of the Society as the National Consultant and Coordinator of the Reach to Recovery Program of the American Cancer Society. I was gratified that the high standards for Volunteers' training established by us were to be maintained and constantly improved.

There are now three categories of Volunteers in the American Cancer Society's Reach to Recovery Program: Women whose duties call for working directly with the patient; women whose duties are in other areas of the Program; and a more recent development, men who help in our Husband-to-Husband Program.

The Volunteer in the first category, who deals personally and directly with the patient, must herself have had a mastectomy.

She is part of this new team effort of doctor, nurse, physiotherapist and patient, which is aimed at attaining the patient's maximum physical and emotional recovery. To be a part of this team requires a very particular temperament and poise. Wanting to help is basic, of course, but that alone is not sufficient. Usually we find that the best of these volunteers are women recommended by surgeons and hospital personnel who, having treated them, are in the ideal position to judge whether they are equipped for the task ahead.

A special effort is made to recruit women who can fit into appropriate "age groups," because a patient will usually identify more readily with, and trust more quickly, a woman of her own age than one who is noticeably older, or younger. For the same reason—gaining a patient's confidence—volunteers are recruited from many ethnic groups.

The Volunteer whose duties are in other areas of the Program is no less essential to Reach to Recovery. Many of these

Volunteers have not had a mastectomy, or for that matter any operation. Among their duties are:

To shop for competent fitters of prosthetic devices in the community and to determine which stores carry which breast forms.

To shop for bathing suits from lists provided by the Reach to Recovery Program, determining which local stores stock which suits and thus spare a new patient this tiring chore.

To visit women's clubs, nursing schools, doctors groups in hospitals, to really make them aware of the Program and its aims.

To assist in the making and assembling of our kits.

To maintain a Telephone Committee, so essential to smooth and efficient functioning of Volunteers as a group.

To supervise training, when qualified, of new Volunteers.

The category of Husband-to-Husband Volunteers originated with the men themselves. Having firsthand knowledge of the husband's role in this situation, they, too, wanted to help. A man whose wife has had a mastectomy—who, himself, has come through the ordeal of doubt and adjustment and helped his wife come through it—is often qualified to counsel and encourage another man about to face the same experience.

Whatever the category of Volunteers, Reach to Recovery has made its application form as simple as possible. There are only four questions to be answered: What, if any, is the applicant's special volunteer training? Previous volunteer experience? Personal health data? Educational background? Formal schooling, by the way, is far less important than understanding and intelligence, a sincere desire to help, and that beautiful quality, compassion. As one of our Volunteers expressed it: "When we make a visit, are we not saying, We love you. We understand—and no strings attached"? That to my mind is compassion, and it is basic to our volunteer approach. The Volunteer who will deal directly with the patient is, in addition, asked to provide the date of her surgery, the hospital where it was performed, her surgeon's and her physician's names and addresses and their approval of her being able, physically and *emotionally,* to undertake this work.

Many outstanding Volunteers have joined the Society's Reach to Recovery Program after hearing about it through newspapers, magazines, films, leaflets, or person-to-person exchange—or from seeing one of the Volunteers interviewed on TV, or hearing one on radio, or through women's clubs, church groups, hospital auxiliaries, or referral by one of the American Cancer Society's other service programs.

There are so many ways a woman can become a part of Reach to Recovery, and in so many cases the volunteer has gone on to become much more involved than she ever dreamed she would be.

One of our Volunteers, reviewing her six years with Reach to Recovery, wrote me: "After having had a mastectomy in October 1963, I heard you speak to nurses at two hospitals in our city in March 1964. Since I am a graduate nurse as well as a mastectomy patient, I recognized the need for such a program and went to work. I was successful in getting the program approved in the hospital where I was operated and visited the first patient there in June 1964. The work soon became a full-time Volunteer job. In the six years since I began with Reach to Recovery I have initiated the Program in 14 hospitals, visited 320 patients in hospitals, more than 50 outside hospitals and offered help and encouragement by phone to many more."

For other Volunteers the route was not at first easy. As one of our most effective workers reminded me: "My dear husband brought me to New York especially to see you because I was still so terribly upset eighteen months following my surgery." That woman, now a Division Coordinator for Reach to Recovery, reported recently: "The state is almost completely organized, and I am delighted. For me it has been like watching a baby grow—some aggravation, a bit of joy and much fulfillment."

Another Volunteer relates that six weeks after her surgery in 1959 she came to work in "my closet." Yes, the quarters were small and crowded in those early days, but the spirit was wonderful. We all knew there was so much to be done—and we pitched in and did it. As this same Volunteer admits, "After much hesitancy on my part in visiting in the hospitals, I must confess these have been the happiest moments of my work with R. to R."

The same echoes of happiness and fulfillment are expressed by so many of our Volunteers. A New Yorker writes: "No other work I have done in all my life has been as rewarding." An Ohio Volunteer puts it this way: "It has given me an opportunity to grow and use some of the talents I never knew existed." And a busy mother and grandmother in Maine wishes she could stretch her days so she could "devote twenty-four hours a day to this great program. And couldn't one go on and on about all the interesting people we meet?"

Indeed one could go on and on. And I wouldn't know where to start or stop in telling about interesting and kind and generous people among our Volunteers. As an example, a recent report from Missouri told me of an endowment established by a Volunteer to provide permanent prostheses "for any woman at our hospital who cannot financially afford to be fitted properly." This thoughtful consideration for others is approached in another way by a Kansas Volunteer who gives lessons to mastectomy patients in how to make their own bras. "Ladies come from a fifty-mile radius to these lessons," she reports proudly.

Another Volunteer from Long Island says: "My first work (in 1959) was to shop the various stores in my part of Long Island to see how well R. to R. patients were treated." Such helpful work, behind the scenes, so to speak, is duplicated all over the country by devoted women—many of them not mastectomy patients—who locate shopping sources, work in Reach to Recovery offices and do the thousand and one necessary tasks that keep the organization running smoothly and effectively.

Over the years I have spoken to many groups of hospital nurses, and I have been deeply impressed by the warm response of the nurses as I have tried to present the special needs of the mastectomy patient, especially the need for understanding on a woman-to-woman basis. Among our Reach to Recovery Volunteers are a number of these nurses, who have not themselves had mastectomies but who bring a special understanding to the situation because of their professional knowledge combined with human sensitivity.

Recently when I was speaking to hospital personnel—any interested hospital employee may attend these talks—I noticed a group of young laboratory technicians in the audience. There were five of these young women, and they sat through the talk I gave several times as other members of the audience arrived and departed. When I was preparing to leave, the five girls came to me all together. Could they become Reach to Recovery Volunteers, they asked, even though they had not had mastectomies? Of course they could, I told them. Curious, I asked them what had prompted this offer to help us. They said that they often had to analyze tissue from mastectomy patients when it was sent to the lab, and now for the first time they realized the human problems faced by the mastectomy patient. She had become a warm human being to them. My heart was warmed by their very human reaction.

I could tell many more stories about our marvelous Volunteers. I have the good fortune to see many of them in my travels about the country. But we have grown beyond that early cozy stage when we all knew each other like family members. I am sometimes a little wistful for the old days, but I am happy about the present and hopeful about the future. As a Volunteer from West Virginia wrote me recently: "How proud and gratified you must be that your program has grown to such proportions."

Indeed I am proud, and each and every Volunteer deserves mention here for her dedication and service.

Space allows specific mention only of those who were the first to volunteer in their county or state—in New York City, Mrs. Walter Rosenau, my wonderful first Volunteer and associate; Mrs. David Sheldon, our second great Volunteer and associate; Mrs. Edward McSweeney, Jr., our third Volunteer, my dear friend and mentor. Joyce Hart from Jamaica, B.W.I., my secretary and dear friend (a real treasure especially in our early days). Mrs. Lou Finkelstein from Brooklyn, devoted keeper of our accounts. From the Bronx, Mrs. Miriam Leal; from Queens, Mrs. Rose Prum; from Brooklyn, Mrs. Renee Levine; from Nassau, Mrs. Ruth Saks; from Suffolk County,

Mrs. Pauline Black; in Albany, New York, Mrs. Emanuel Weil.

And in New Jersey, Bea Hutner, Mrs. Edgar Warner and Eleanor Mordwin; in Maryland, Sonia Lowitz; in San Francisco, Rhoda Goldman and in Los Angeles, Mrs. Anita Rogers Douglas; in Connecticut, Helen Loth; in Florida, Madeleine RossKam; in Pennsylvania, Dale Boyd; in Detroit, Annette Rosen.

And in Ohio, Helen Moyer and Mrs. David Moore (both non-mastectomy Volunteers), Pauly Oldham, Shirley Sheldon (ACS Cleveland Coordinator), Dorothy Weber (State Coordinator, non-mastectomy Volunteer, since 1954); in Tennessee, Dodie Allman; in Kentucky, Dorothy Duncan; in Wisconsin, Mrs. Richard D. Wolfgrams; in Georgia, Mildred Durden; in Minnesota, Mrs. C. Poppenberger (these last three all non-mastectomy Volunteers).

And in Pennsylvania, Sylvia Schuster; in Virginia, Adice Waymack; in West Virginia, Bea Kleeman and Calvert Jones; in Mississippi, Margaret May (a non-mastectomy Volunteer); in Maine, Barbara Lynch; in Missouri, Mrs. Gunther Schmidt (a non-mastectomy Volunteer) and in Kansas, Mrs. Ernest Robinson.

And so many other wonderful Volunteers, too numerous to mention, who are still the backbone of the Program and to whom I want always to give heartfelt thanks.

What a blessing, indeed, that the concern about cancer cuts across the turbulence of our era like a streak of sanity and human compassion!

Imagine for a moment that now you, yourself, wish to become an American Cancer Society Reach to Recovery Volunteer.

You have filled out the application form, and your surgeon and your physician have approved your service as a Volunteer.

What comes next?

Appearance counts in qualifying for the Program; this is not to say that you need dress expensively or in the latest fashion. Not at all. But you should be well groomed. Your posture should be good. Your figure must be centered (Chapter VI) and your prosthesis well fitted. It is also necessary that you have complete movement of both arms. Personality counts, too—project optimism and self-confidence, and you provide visible evidence of your adjustment to your own operation, emotionally as well as physically.

Having qualified both in appearance and personality to work directly with the patient, you are screened by the local American Cancer Society unit and indoctrinated in our code of ethics. A Reach to Recovery trainer then begins your training.

All decisions about exercises, all answers to medical questions, are referred to the patient's doctor.

The trainee—you—will be given a detailed analysis, with actual samples, of the various prosthetic forms shown by *Reach to Recovery,* told why these particular forms are shown, and instructed in how to counsel a patient about securing a proper fitting.

(These sample breast forms, by the way, always accompany me on a lecture trip abroad. They are in an impressive range of shapes and sizes. One customs inspector in South America was especially impressed. Opening my bags, he gaped, choked, then said in a hushed tone, "Señora, these are yours, personally?" "Oh, yes." "*All* of them, yours, personally?" "All of them." A more detailed explanation might have been given but the man was already signalling other inspectors to come have a look. There was a unanimous shaking of masculine heads. "Women! Who can understand them? Especially these crazy Americans!")

Having familiarized yourself with our prostheses, you are next instructed about the Kit—how to pack one, your responsibility for its care and safekeeping, and how to unpack it in a patient's presence; how to dry a breast form (in time you will be called upon to demonstrate this); how to make an underarm roll and a support sling (Chapter II); how to teach exercises.

Your training will also include indoctrination on advising a patient on bras and clothing, lounge bras and swimsuits, and how to center and dress her figure.

In short, a trainee is thoroughly grounded in the use of every tool of rehabilitation provided by the Reach to Recovery Program *before being trained in the various approaches to the patient in person.* A Volunteer's initial meeting with a patient is always important, sometimes quite delicate, and as a trainee you are supplied with a Reach to Recovery booklet, *Suggestions for Visiting the Patient,* which is most helpful in this regard. It contains guidance covering the following points:

1. Making certain your visit is always approved by the attending physician.
2. Being informed, prior to meeting the patient, about certain data about her (bra size; Is she married? Can she be given exercises?).
3. Checking your own grooming in the nearest ladies' room, to be sure you look your attractive best when the patient sees you for the first time.

4. Introducing yourself to the patient—how to act, what to do and say to establish rapport.
5. Opening the Kit to show, first, the *Manual,* which contains your name and phone number to provide access to continuing help if a patient needs it.
6. Demonstrating the use of the rubber ball on elastic string, how to start exercising with it, and how to increase the exercise.
7. Demonstrating wall climbing, explaining its purpose, assisting the patient to do this exercise herself.
8. Demonstrating how to use the plastic-coated rope as a pulley, then as an aid for doing circular exercises with the arm on the side of the operation.
9. Showing the patient, in front of a mirror, correct posture and how to square off her shoulders.
10. Demonstrating how to carry an object of some weight, such as a large purse, a package, or a child.
11. Showing the patient how to walk well and how to relax.

The booklet also covers what a Volunteer should say—*and should not say*—on the subject of the patient's adjustment to husband, family and friends when she returns home.

The time required to train a Volunteer is usually two full days. Should you, as a trainee, show a special empathy for the work and decide to undertake a larger role in the Program, your training would of course be more extensive.

No one type of personality is especially suited to work as a Volunteer in the Society's Reach to Recovery Program. Women of all races with whom I had the privilege of working in South Africa provided particularly graphic evidence of this.

Via London, Zurich, and Nairobi, I arrived in Johannesburg to be most warmly greeted by members of the National Cancer Association of South Africa and a surprisingly large turnout of representatives of the press and radio reporters with tape recorders. These latter gentlemen had done their homework! Their questioning showed not only an understanding of my mission (which was, in part, to train Volunteers) but an intelligent and sympathetic interest in it, and in the entire international movement toward rehabilitation of the cancer patient.

At the conclusion of the interview I announced that all women who had had a mastectomy were invited to come—and bring their husbands—to the auditorium of the Institute of Medical Research the following evening at eight, when I was scheduled to lecture. Prior to this trip I had been advised that attendance at this lecture would be restricted to professional people, fifty in all, admittance to be by written invitation only. When I suggested that women who had undergone mastectomy would also benefit by attending, the answer was, "You must understand that women here are not like women in the United States. By tradition and background they are much more reticent. None would come to such a meeting and be identified by others in the community."

But this had not proven to be so elsewhere outside the U.S. Why should women in Johannesburg be so different from women the world over? Thus my somewhat unexpected public invitation—if these women felt the Reach to Recovery Program could help them, let them come and be helped!

Reservations had been made for me at the pleasant Casa Mia Hotel. I went there from the airport, and straight up to my room, aching to get out of my travel-rumpled clothes and into a hot tub. While the water was running, the phone rang.

Ten minutes later, still talking on the phone about certain minor rearrangements in my schedule for the next thirty-six hours, I heard an odd gurgling sound and glanced toward the bathroom. The tub had overflowed. A veritable river was pouring into the bedroom. Before I could get to the tub and turn the taps, I was sloshing ankle-deep in steaming water.

In retrospect the incident seems amusing. At the time it assuredly was not—because I discovered that no other room could possibly be made available until the next morning . . .

The auditorium at the Institute of Medical Research was located on the ground floor in a parklike garden. Two hours before the hour set for the lecture, I arrived to find the place entirely filled except for the fifty seats reserved for those special guests bearing written invitations. And people were still clamoring to get in. Women, indeed, *are* women the world over! Many had taken my suggestion and brought their husbands along, too.

While members of the Association hastily began setting up chairs outside the open windows, I requested the men seated in the audience to give up their chairs to women. A few obligingly did so. Most stayed put. Finally, by placing additional chairs in open doorways, everyone was accommodated.

Altogether it was a memorable occasion. So was my entire tour of South Africa. The coverage given Reach to Recovery by the media was more than generous. Newspapers not only carried feature articles about the Program but also front-page stories about it. Radio stations accorded it prime time special-feature treatment. By the time I reached Capetown, women were coming from as far away as Durban, hundreds of miles distant. Again and again, those words from the earliest days of the Program were echoed: "I only wish I had had someone to come and talk to me when I was in the hospital. May I be of help?"

They were not words spoken idly by these women. Many were away from their homes for the first time in their lives. And they had journeyed to Capetown prepared to remain for as long as it took them to be trained as Reach to Recovery Volunteers—and carry back with them, to their distant homes, help for other women in the same situation. The country now has a fine Reach to Recovery Program.

At a meeting of the American Cancer Society's National Service Committee, a distinguished surgeon summed up very well the effect that a Reach to Recovery Volunteer has upon a mastectomy patient. Referring to radical surgery he had performed on a forty-five-year-old woman, the speaker said the operation had been highly successful with a prognosis of complete control, and that the patient was so informed.

Despite this encouragement, the woman was "emotionally unglued." The surgeon said, "It was then that I asked her if she would like to talk to one of our Reach to Recovery Volunteers who had had a similar operation. She eagerly agreed and a phone call brought a Volunteer to her bedside. The enthusiasm of this attractive young woman, with the message she brought to this downcast patient, effected a tremendous change in outlook. The Volunteer was able to answer questions that patients rarely ask of surgeons. The confidence generated has significant healing qualities."

What a glow of satisfaction, warmed by humility, to be in a position of conveying to someone in deep distress "significant healing qualities," to see despair turn to hope in their eyes!

A final word about you yourself becoming an ACS Reach to Recovery Volunteer: You may work only a few hours a week, visiting one hospital a few city blocks from your home, or you may work many hours and cross hundreds of miles of open country visiting hospitals county-wide—including, as one Volunteer does, visiting an Indian Reservation. The choice is yours. The requirement is a desire to help women help themselves to recover, physically and mentally, from a mastectomy.

A woman came up after a meeting in Kansas City and asked if she might have a word with me privately. She was middle-aged, quite pretty, and wore an ankle-length mink coat and a very smart matching mink hat.

We moved to a corner of the stage and stepped behind a screen.

"You should know," she said quietly, "that you have just saved my life."

A figure of speech, I thought, and smiled, waiting for her to go on to whatever it was she wished to discuss.

"Five months ago," she said, "I had a radical mastectomy. Since then, nothing has been right. I've been depressed, my husband's been miserable. It's reached a point where I hate to wake up in the morning knowing I must live through another day of utter wretchedness." She opened her purse. "So I made up my mind to put an end to it."

She held out her hand. In it was a bottle of sleeping pills.

My smile vanished.

"I walked into this meeting," she went on, "certain that I would walk out of it, go home, and take these." She drew a long breath, closed her fingers about the bottle of pills and shoved her hands deep into her coat pockets. "Only I didn't walk out. I stayed, and listened."

"And I hope changed your mind!"

"I've decided that kind of thinking was plain stupidity."

Now it was she who managed a smile. "I have my share of failings," she said softly, drawing her fur snugly about her, "but one I do not have is plain stupidity. I want to thank you for reminding me of that."

How often a woman's deepest heartache is never put into words—and even so, how often Reach to Recovery's message from woman to woman has been able to touch the heartache and ease it!

As a Volunteer, you will carry that message. There are few experiences in your life that will be more rewarding.

X

Tomorrow, and Tomorrow . . .

Our doubts are traitors,
And make us lose the good we oft might win,
By fearing to attempt.
—William Shakespeare

There was a time when doubts were inevitable to a woman who underwent a mastectomy. In 1900, the cure rate for all types of cancer was only one in seven. Today, when localized breast cancer has the encouraging cure rate of 85 percent, and every effort is being made to better that rate, the woman who fears to attempt a maximum effort at recovery is betraying her most precious commodity—herself.

It is your own *will to recover* that is the key to your future following a mastectomy. Without that will, that determination on your part, the team effort in your behalf by doctor, nurse, physiotherapist and Reach to Recovery Volunteer has slight chance of succeeding.

A noted specialist, speaking at an ACS-sponsored meeting, declared that "Survival in itself is not enough for anyone. To live successfully, a person must find constructive ways of controlling fears and anxieties, experience satisfactions in the activities of the day and have confidence in her ability to handle the challenges of the future. To help an individual achieve these goals is the mission of total rehabilitation."

A co-worker in the Reach to Recovery Program had a small grandchild who was struggling to pronounce that word "rehabilitation." For a five-year-old, it was a formidable challenge.

"You keep missing those two syllables," the grandmother corrected patiently. "What you're saying, dear, comes out sounding like 'revelation.' "

And so it did, missing those two syllables—but the thought crossed my mind, *There really isn't much difference when you stop to think about it,* because rehabilitation means the restoring of health and efficiency, and when it's successful it *is* a revelation—of the human spirit's indomitable capacity for triumphing over anxieties, fears, and the dark specter of defeat.

Here at the American Cancer Society we have witnessed many such triumphs. The exception—defeat instead of victory—too often occurs when panic warps a woman's judgment and common sense, as it did Vivian F.'s.

Setting up for a meeting in Jackson, Mississippi, I noted a young man in the second row with a tape recorder. He came forward, introduced himself as a minister from one of the nearby churches, and asked whether he might tape the lecture.

"Of course. But why, may I ask?"

He explained that he was often called upon to counsel women who had had breast surgery. "A tape of your lecture will make up for my inadequacies to do that." He added that he'd brought along two members of his parish who very much needed counseling; would I speak with them, in private, before the meeting got under way?

The younger of the two women, Mrs. O'M., had returned home from the hospital only the day before. When the minister had urged her to accompany him to this meeting she had protested that she was not yet strong enough to go out.

"I told her," the minister said, placing a hand gently on her shoulder, "that if I had to put her on a stretcher and have her carried in, she would be here."

Mrs. O'M. managed a pale smile. "He was right, as usual," she said. "I can always rest, but I can't always have this."

The minister introduced the other woman as Vivian F.

"I'm a patient of Dr. C.'s" Vivian told me. "Perhaps you know of him?"

Most of the hospital's surgeons were known to me by name, but I could not recall having heard of Dr. C.

Vivian explained that he was not a surgeon, nor was he on the hospital's staff. "I had been going to Dr. McD.," she went on, "until I discovered a lump in my breast and he wanted to do a biopsy and, if necessary, a mastectomy. Then I just panicked."

Dr. McD. was the chief of surgery, whom I knew well. In his hands there was no need for Vivian to panic, and I urged her by all means to follow his advice.

She shook her head. "I'm not his patient any more," she said. "You see, my wonderful Dr. C. says there's no reason I have to have an operation at all, ever."

A chill raced down my spine. I began to suspect why Dr. C. was not on the hospital's staff. A glance at the minister was enough to confirm my suspicions; he nodded grimly.

I asked Vivian exactly what Dr. C. did recommend.

She smiled. "Just a simple series of treatments."

What sort of treatments?

"He calls them temperature-ray infusions."

And what, exactly, were "temperature-ray infusions"?

"Well," Vivian said, "he gives them right in his office, with this perfectly marvelous machine he has there. It's his own invention." Beyond that, her explanation was vague. She would be visiting Dr. C.'s office three times a week for a period of six months. On each visit, seated before the machine, heat and cold were alternated upon the area of her breast where the lump was. Each treatment lasted fifteen minutes. It left no disfigurement, and was entirely painless. "And," Vivian concluded firmly, "Dr. C. absolutely guarantees a cure!"

Later the minister told me that he had brought this woman to the meeting hoping to persuade her to return to the care of Dr. McD. "Six months in C.'s hands and it might be too late! I thought if she could see for herself that losing a breast isn't the end of the world for a woman, her fear of surgery would subside enough so she'd listen to reason."

Perhaps it should not be surprising when a frightened woman turns from sobering reality to such fantasies of wishful thinking as a "guaranteed cure" for cancer—but it *is* tragic. Time is lost—precious, irreplaceable time—just when early diagnosis and effective treatment could conquer the disease. And discouragement is doubly acute when the patient discovers—as, inevitably and cruelly, she does discover—that the guarantee is worthless.

The toll in suffering and death from such promises of nonexistent cures is incalculable.

"The patient who allows her cancer to become advanced while seeking or trying a worthless remedy," the American Cancer Society warns, "is in greatest peril." When a cell in the body undergoes a change and becomes malignant, it reproduces itself by division, two cells dividing to become four, those four then dividing to become eight, those eight becoming sixteen, on and on and on—and all descendants of the original cell are themselves equally malignant. The earlier that cycle of division is halted, the fewer cells will have been reproduced; the less chance for the cancer to spread, the better the body can regain robust good health.

Because there is no greater initial service to perform for the patient than to achieve such early diagnosis, the American Cancer Society initiated in 1969 its Clinical Investigation Program to speed the latest scientific findings to the patient—and thus combat with truth the empty promises of Dr. C. and his kind. Also, the Professional Education Department of the Society maintains a section on Unproved Methods of Cancer Management which, in a single twelve-month period, added more than 4,000 items to its files on unproven methods of treatment, handled many hundreds of requests for information, and distributed informative statements to the 58 divisions of the Society, to science writers, and to physicians.

Even so, news of the latest "miracle cure" spreads like a brushfire, and the quack continues to thrive, with an incredible word-of-mouth neighborhood communication network operating in his behalf.

To many people, the word "cancer" is still so overwhelming that, like Vivian F., they tragically—and unnecessarily—panic and rush headlong to some charlatan who, in fact, can offer only one guarantee: that the cost of his "miracle cure" will be high.

Its cost, too often, is life itself.

In Jackson that afternoon, before the meeting was started, I was able to fit Mrs. O'M. with a breast form that brought a sparkle to her eyes and a new air of confidence to her manner. She remained, with her pastor, until the meeting was over.

Vivian F. did not.

The moment I urged her to heed her surgeon's advice, she lost interest in anything I had to say. Watching her turn and go slowly up the aisle of the auditorium, I was reminded of the ACS television film on quackery, "Journey Into Darkness." Its closing scene is most poignant, with a group of people as misguided as Vivian F., entering an airport tunnel for a flight into the shadows of false hopes and futility.

Considerable time passed before I had occasion to be in Jackson again. One of the first things I did was telephone the minister to inquire about Vivian F.

There was a moment's silence before he replied.

"Vivian became disenchanted with C. and his machine," the minister said, "and was finally prepared to face up to surgery." Again, a moment of silence. "But by then she had waited too long," he said quietly, "and it was just too late."

In his State of the Union message as this nation entered the decade of the Seventies, President Nixon said, "The time has come in America when the same kind of concentrated effort that split the atom and took man to the moon should be turned toward conquering this dread disease." The President urged a total national commitment to achieve the conquest of cancer, declaring his intention of providing an extra $100 million immediately in the search for a cure and promising to ask later for whatever additional funds might be used effectively.

So the American Cancer Society's objective of making the Seventies the decade that brings control of cancer within sight is moving closer to attainment. Advances in research and therapy over recent years make the view of the future the most hopeful it has ever been.

But optimism cannot—*must not*—lead to complacency.

"Whatever the achievements in cancer control," a spokesman for the Society has emphasized, "we measure progress against the continuing and tragic toll. . . . All that has happened must be considered prologue to intensified and enlarged programs of cancer control."

And in that same spirit, all that has happened with Reach to Recovery is but prologue to the Society's plans to intensify and enlarge its rehabilitation service to the individual cancer patient.

What a distance has been traveled since that day almost two decades ago when my surgeon said to me, "Do something about it!"—and what a distance there is still to be traveled. In the beginning the journey was solitary, but it is solitary no longer. One unit of a Midwest American Cancer Society division reported that two hospitals averaging per year, together, more than a hundred mastectomies, had a Reach to Recovery Volunteer visit *every mastectomy patient* during a six-month period. An Eastern division reported that four Reach to Recovery Volunteers were assigned to a major teaching hospital *on a permanent basis,* to assist with its post-mastectomy classes. Of all cancer patients assisted with rehabilitation by all Divisions, *more than 56 percent* were mastectomy patients. And a staff member with a tenure of sixteen years with one division has been quoted as saying, "This program [Reach to Recovery] is proving to be the most rewarding of all programs ACS has ever conducted."

So, as you reach to your own recovery, to your own triumph over defeat and despair, know that you are not alone.

Remember that to doubt yourself is to betray yourself—whereas the Reach to Recovery Program is an affirmation of yourself and your indomitable capacity as a woman to achieve your physical and emotional recovery.

Remember, too, that you are not reaching backward to the life you knew before your operation, but forward to a more vigorous, more rewarding and exciting life.

Remember, above all, that to be alive means to *grow*.

You are not less, but can be more a woman than you were before this operation—because our concept of rehabilitation defines "recovery after mastectomy" as *growing to become a better woman*—in every way.

The blessings allotted to you are generous. All that is necessary is to look, to find them.

So until, perhaps, we meet one day in person, may God hold you in the palm of His hand.

EPILOGUE

CANCER of the breast is the most common form of cancer in women today. It is estimated that there will be 71,000 new cases in 1972, and that seven out of every hundred American women will some day develop this disease.

Surgery requiring removal of the breast will be the treatment of choice for the vast majority of these women.

The rehabilitation of this large number of women, scattered throughout the United States, who have had breast surgery presents a problem of major proportions. We have seen how Terese Lasser fought to develop a program to assist these women. We have read of her successes and sensed her frustrations during the early years.

The merger of the Reach to Recovery Program with the American Cancer Society in 1969 brought the vast resources of the Society into play. Now that a national voluntary health agency with strong professional and lay leadership was committed, Reach to Recovery had access at the grass-roots level to the more than 3,000 American Cancer Society Units throughout the country. The program could be brought into the small community hospital as well as the large urban medical center. Ted Lasser's inspired leadership and the technical expertise and the organizational skills of the ACS together created a force that showed great promise.

Our expectations were more than realized. During the first

year (1969–70) of the operation of the Reach to Recovery Program as a Service and Rehabilitation activity of the ACS, 1,825 Volunteers visited and assisted 7,671 women in 952 hospitals. Two thousand nine hundred and seven physicians requested this service for their patients. During the second year, 1970–71, these were the vital statistics: Active Volunteers increased in number to 3,355, and they visited and assisted more than twice as many patients—17,481—in 1,571 hospitals. The number of physicians requesting the service for their patients was 5,694, nearly double the number of physicians who used the Program in 1969–70.

One can only conclude that the concept of a carefully selected and trained mastectomy Volunteer working under medical supervision as a member of the rehabilitation team had won the enthusiastic support of the medical profession. We have every reason to hope that with each passing year the total needs of the mastectomy patient will be more clearly and more widely recognized and successfully met.

Meanwhile we give hearty thanks to Ted Lasser and her devoted Reach to Recovery Volunteers, to the many physicians who have supported and used the Reach to Recovery Program, and to the lay and professional Volunteers and staff at all levels of the ACS, locally and nationally, who are helping make Reach to Recovery available to the woman who has had breast surgery, wherever she may be.

—William M. Markel, M.D.
Vice President for Service
and Rehabilitation
American Cancer Society